T0260014

Evidence in Medicine

Evidence in Medicine

The Common Flaws,
Why They Occur and
How to Prevent Them

Iain K Crombie

University of Dundee
Dundee, Scotland, UK

WILEY Blackwell

This edition first published 2021
© 2021 John Wiley & Sons Ltd

All rights reserved. No part of this publication may be reproduced, stored in a retrieval system, or transmitted, in any form or by any means, electronic, mechanical, photocopying, recording or otherwise, except as permitted by law. Advice on how to obtain permission to reuse material from this title is available at http://www.wiley.com/go/permissions.

The right of Iain K Crombie to be identified as the author of this work has been asserted in accordance with law.

Registered Office(s)
John Wiley & Sons, Inc., 111 River Street, Hoboken, NJ 07030, USA
John Wiley & Sons Ltd, The Atrium, Southern Gate, Chichester, West Sussex, PO19 8SQ, UK

Editorial Office
9600 Garsington Road, Oxford, OX4 2DQ, UK

For details of our global editorial offices, customer services, and more information about Wiley products visit us at www.wiley.com.

Wiley also publishes its books in a variety of electronic formats and by print-on-demand. Some content that appears in standard print versions of this book may not be available in other formats.

Limit of Liability/Disclaimer of Warranty
The contents of this work are intended to further general scientific research, understanding and discussion only and are not intended and should not be relied upon as recommending or promoting scientific method, diagnosis or treatment by physicians for any particular patient. In view of ongoing research, equipment modifications, changes in governmental regulations and the constant flow of information relating to the use of medicines, equipment and devices, the reader is urged to review and evaluate the information provided in the package insert or instructions for each medicine, equipment or device for, among other things, any changes in the instructions or indication of usage and for added warnings and precautions. While the publisher and authors have used their best efforts in preparing this work, they make no representations or warranties with respect to the accuracy or completeness of the contents of this work and specifically disclaim all warranties, including without limitation any implied warranties of merchantability or fitness for a particular purpose. No warranty may be created or extended by sales representatives, written sales materials or promotional statements for this work. The fact that an organisation, website or product is referred to in this work as a citation and/or potential source of further information does not mean that the publisher and authors endorse the information or services the organisation, website or product may provide or recommendations it may make. This work is sold with the understanding that the publisher is not engaged in rendering professional services. The advice and strategies contained herein may not be suitable for your situation. You should consult with a specialist where appropriate. Further, readers should be aware that websites listed in this work may have changed or disappeared between when this work was written and when it is read. Neither the publisher nor authors shall be liable for any loss of profit or any other commercial damages, including but not limited to special, incidental, consequential or other damages.

Library of Congress Cataloging-in-Publication Data

Names: Crombie, I. K., author.
Title: Evidence in medicine : the common flaws, why they occur and how to
   prevent them / Iain K. Crombie.
Description: First edition. | Hoboken, NJ : John Wiley & Sons, Inc., 2021.
   | Includes bibliographical references and index.
Identifiers: LCCN 2020051750 (print) | LCCN 2020051751 (ebook) | ISBN
   9781119794141 (paperback) | ISBN 9781119794189 (adobe pdf) | ISBN
   9781119794196 (epub)
Subjects: MESH: Research Design–standards | Randomized Controlled Trials
   as Topic | Systematic Reviews as Topic | Evidence-Based
   Practice–standards | Treatment Outcome
Classification: LCC R852 (print) | LCC R852 (ebook) | NLM W 20.5 | DDC
   610.72–dc23
LC record available at https://lccn.loc.gov/2020051750
LC ebook record available at https://lccn.loc.gov/2020051751

Cover Design: Wiley
Cover Image: © Govindanmarudhai/DigitalVision Vectors/Getty Images

Set in 10.5/13pt STIXTwoText by SPi Global, Pondicherry, India
Printed and bound by CPI Group (UK) Ltd, Croydon, CR0 4YY

C9781119794141_060421

Contents

Preface

Evidence is central to the practice of medicine. The amount of published medical evidence is immense, but there are widespread concerns about the quality of many studies. Deficiencies in the conduct of research studies often result in misleading estimates of the benefits of treatments, so that ineffective treatments may be used in clinical practice. In addition, many studies are wasted because they have been so poorly designed and conducted.

This book explores the nature of the deficiencies and flaws in the evidence about the effectiveness of treatments. It is the result of a career-long interest in medical evidence. A recent career change provided an opportunity to read the extensive literature on research quality that has emerged in recent years. As befits a book on evidence, references are cited to support the statements made. Reviews and commentaries are used where available, although many landmark studies are also referenced. The approach taken is to cite sufficient papers to support a point, rather than give a comprehensive a review of it. The number of references cited reflect the wealth of evidence on the deficiencies in medical research.

I am grateful to the University of Dundee for providing the facilities to research and write this book, and to my colleagues for their support and encouragement. Special thanks are due to my long-time colleague and friend Linda Irvine: she made several gently delivered, trenchant criticisms of early drafts and picked out factual, logical and grammatical failings in later drafts. The irony of writing a book about evidence is that it may contain errors of fact or interpretation. Equally there may be errors of omission. I take full responsibility for all flaws.

Aims of this Book

The advent of the randomised controlled trial (RCT) provided a method to generate reliable evidence on the effectiveness of treatments. It enables a fair comparison of groups [1], and should identify which treatments are beneficial and which are of little or no value. Since the early randomised controlled trials (RCTs) of the mid-twentieth century, the design of trials has been progressively refined, making them the bedrock on which modern medicine is built. The findings of RCTs are used by regulatory authorities across the world to licence effective treatments. Other methods of testing treatments have been proposed, but none matches the ability of high quality randomised trials to provide good estimates of treatment effectiveness [2]. The RCT deserves its status as the gold standard for assessing the effectiveness of treatment.

The RCT now occupies a leading place in medical research, with tens of thousands of trials being published annually [3, 4]. These studies should provide high quality evidence across all fields of medicine, but that promise has not been fulfilled. At issue is the quality of the evidence. Concerns are growing 'about the reliability and validity of the underlying research that supports regulatory and clinical decision-making' [5], with authors describing 'the pervasiveness of poor quality clinical evidence' [6] and concluding that 'much of the published medical research is apparently flawed, cannot be replicated and/or has limited or no utility' [7]. In a particularly trenchant comment, Ian Roberts and colleagues concluded that 'the knowledge system underpinning healthcare is not fit for purpose and must change' [8]. This book evaluates that proposition.

To investigate the knowledge system for healthcare, this book poses five questions: 1) what are the problems; 2) how common are they; 3) to what extent do they bias evidence; 4) why do they occur, and 5) how can they be prevented? Medical research is a vast enterprise, so the book focuses on the two most important research methods: the randomised controlled trial and the systematic review. Answers to the first three questions will provide a broad assessment of the quality of evidence (Chapters 2–5). The answer to the fourth question, on the causes of poor quality, highlights issues around misconduct and how the structures and incentives in the research environment influence the quality of evidence (Chapters 6 and 7). The final chapter presents an approach for developing a comprehensive strategy to the quality problem. This is supported by an Appendix, which lists the initiatives that have been proposed to improve research evidence. First, to introduce the nature of evidence in medicine, Chapter 1 provides a brief review of the rationale for treatments from ancient times to the present day.

This book focuses on the flaws in medical evidence. It does not review the important findings from the many high quality studies that have provided convincing evidence on the effectiveness of a wide range of treatments. Instead, the book describes the variety of deficiencies that afflict much research. This assessment could lead to an overly negative assessment of the state of medical evidence. The reality is that clinical research is spread across a spectrum from high to very low quality studies. The aim of the book is to use a detailed review of the flaws and their causes, to develop a strategy to prevent poor quality and misleading research. If implemented, the strategy could prevent some of the more egregious studies from being published, and rectify some with less reprehensible weaknesses. In this way, it could help move the spectrum upwards in quality. The book should be read from a constructive perspective of what is going wrong and how can we change it, in which the focus on flaws also provides the motivation for action.

REFERENCES

1. Chalmers, I. (2011). Why the 1948 MRC trial of streptomycin used treatment allocation based on random numbers. *J. R. Soc. Med.* 104: 383–386.
2. Byar, D.P., Simon, R.M., Friedewald, W.T. et al. (1976). Randomized clinical trials. Perspectives on some recent ideas. *N. Engl. J. Med.* 295: 74–80.

3. Bastian, H., Glasziou, P., and Chalmers, I. (2010). Seventy-five trials and eleven systematic reviews a day: how will we ever keep up? *PLoS Med.* https://doi.org/10.1371/journal.pmed.1000326.

4. Viergever, R.F. and Li, K. (2015). Trends in global clinical trial registration: an analysis of numbers of registered clinical trials in different parts of the world from 2004 to 2013. *BMJ Open* https://doi.org/10.1136/bmjopen-2015-008932.

5. Wallach, J.D., Gonsalves, G.S., and Ross, J.S. (2018). Research, regulatory, and clinical decision-making: the importance of scientific integrity. *J. Clin. Epidemiol.* 93: 88–93.

6. Ioannidis, J.P.A., Stuart, M.E., Brownlee, S. et al. (2017). How to survive the medical misinformation mess. *Eur. J. Clin. Investig.* 47: 795–802.

7. Eshre, C.W.G. (2018). Protect us from poor-quality medical research. *Hum. Reprod.* 33: 770–776.

8. Roberts, I., Ker, K., Edwards, P. et al. (2015). The knowledge system underpinning healthcare is not fit for purpose and must change. *BMJ* https://doi.org/10.1136/bmj.h2463.

CHAPTER 1

The Rationale for Treatment

A Brief History

The development of modern medicine has rightly been described as 'the greatest benefit to mankind' [1]. Vaccination, anaesthetics, aseptic surgery, antibiotics, insulin for diabetes and drugs to prevent and treat heart disease form part of a very long list of treatments that have transformed healthcare. These are the fruits of many years of careful clinical investigation supported by extensive research. However, medicine has a checkered history in which ineffective treatments were widely used: as Benjamin Franklin pithily remarked in the eighteenth century, 'God heals, and the doctor takes the fees' [2]. Studies of the history of medicine show that the basis on which treatments have been used has varied greatly across the centuries [3]. This chapter explores the rationale behind the use of treatments, and the way this

Evidence in Medicine: The Common Flaws, Why They Occur and How to Prevent Them, First Edition. Iain K Crombie.
© 2021 John Wiley & Sons Ltd. Published 2021 by John Wiley & Sons Ltd.

has changed over time. It concludes by describing the progress towards present-day methods for testing the effectiveness of treatments.

THEORY AS JUSTIFICATION FOR TREATMENT

In ancient times diseases were attributed to supernatural causes, spirits and demons. Treatments involved spells and prayers, or the wearing of amulets, which were intended to drive the malign forces from the patient [4]. Theories gradually evolved towards biological and physical causes of disease, with treatments involving minor surgery and drugs (usually based on plant extracts, minerals and metals). In Western medicine, one of the most influential of these theories was the doctrine of the four humours. It held that good health was enjoyed when four humours (the fluids: blood, phlegm, black bile and yellow bile) were in balance, with an excess of one humour causing disease [5]. Treatment for illness focused on restoring the balance by removing some of the excess humour from the body. This could be achieved by bloodletting (cutting open a vein or by applying a leech), or by losing fluid with a purgative or blistering the skin. This treatment was almost always harmful, although it often appeared to give short-term relief of the symptoms of acute inflammations [6]. The most notable casualty of bloodletting was George Washington, first president of the United States. He was suffering from a serious upper respiratory tract infection, for which his doctors extracted approximately 2.4 L of blood over about 12 hours. He died 33 hours later, probably from the combination of the infection and the treatment given [5]. When the practice of bloodletting was challenged in the nineteenth century, a leading physician, William Stokes, commented that it was hard to believe 'that the fathers of British medicine were always in error, and that they were bad observers and mistaken practitioners' [7]. This cautionary tale of bloodletting suggests that theory and clinical experience may be unreliable guides to the effectiveness of a treatment.

A more recent but widely (mis)used theory was that bed rest was beneficial for a variety of ailments. Its popularity has been traced to a series of lectures in the middle nineteenth century by

John Hilton, president of the Royal College of Surgeons [8, 9]. Initially recommended for recovery following orthopaedic procedures [10], it was soon used for conditions including myocardial infarction, pulmonary tuberculosis, rheumatic fever and psychiatric illnesses [9]. Bed rest was particularly popular in pregnancy, where it was recommended for complications such as threatened abortion, hypertension or preterm labour [11]. The theory was that if rest helped to mend broken bones, then it would also heal other organs [9]. The benefits of bed rest were thought to include reduced demands on the heart, conservation of metabolic resources for healing and avoidance of stress [12]. Its use began to be challenged in the middle of the twentieth century, as evidence grew on the adverse effects of bed rest; it is now known to cause impairment of cardiovascular, haematological, musculoskeletal, immune and psychological functions [9, 12]. Bed rest is an example of a treatment based on beliefs about benefit that endured in the face of substantial evidence of harm [8, 11].

TESTING ON A SERIES OF PATIENTS

The transition, from treatments based on theory to the use of evidence derived from empirical studies, was a gradual process. A simple, and common, method was to give a treatment on a series of patients, then observe its impact on disease. A good example is the use of the leaves of the willow tree for inflamed joints, a treatment dating back to the ancient Egyptians [13]. Clinical observation confirmed the benefits: application of a decoction of willow leaves to inflamed skin reduced the swelling. Extracts of willow leaves and bark were also used for fever and pain by the Greeks from the fifth century BCE [14]. An important step in the use of the willow was taken by the Reverend Edward Stone in 1763. He administered a solution of powdered willow bark to 50 patients with fever, judging the treatment a great success [14, 15]. The active ingredient of the willow, salicin, was isolated in the 1820s [13, 15]. This drug was tested by a Dundee physician, T.J. MacLagan, who administered it to a series of patients with acute rheumatism. Not only was the treatment successful, it demonstrated antipyretic, analgesic and anti-inflammatory effects [15]. Salicin was recognised to be an important drug, but its long-term use was limited because gastric irritation, nausea and vomiting were common side effects. The pharmaceutical arm of the Bayer company searched for a safer alternative, and successfully modified salicin to produce a new chemical with fewer side effects [13, 15]. That drug, aspirin, is now the most widely used medicine in the world [14].

Another example of evidence from a series of patients is the discovery of insulin for the treatment of diabetes. This was undoubtedly 'one of the most dramatic events in the history of the treatment of disease' [16]. Research, in the late nineteenth century, had shown that removal of an animal's pancreas 'produced severe and fatal diabetes' [17]. Over the following 30 years many researchers tried to isolate a pancreatic extract that could control blood sugar levels. They had little success, as the extracts had only a transitory effect on blood sugar and caused unacceptable side effects (vomiting, fever and convulsions) [18, 19]. In October 1920 Frederick Banting, a young Canadian doctor, was preparing a lecture on the pancreas [16]. The research he was reading led him to think that the active ingredient was being destroyed by the digestive enzymes in the pancreas, and that this could be prevented by ligating the pancreatic ducts. Banting began the experiments with extracts of the ligated pancreas in May 1921 [17]. By January 1922 a purified extract had been obtained. This proved successful in treating a 14-year-old boy, and in February a further six patients were treated with equally favourable results [16]. The discovery was announced in April to international acclaim; the Nobel prize was awarded to Banting, and one of his colleagues, Dr Macleod, in 1923 [16].

COMPARING GROUPS

Case series can provide support for a treatment if, as with insulin, the benefits are immediate and substantial. But observations on a set of patients are often not sufficient to identify whether a treatment is truly effective. Consider the management of gunshot wounds in the sixteenth century. At that time it was believed that the bullet introduced poison into the body, and that cauterising the wound with boiling oil mixed with treacle would detoxify it [20, 21]. The treatment was very unpleasant, but was thought to save lives. Force of circumstances led the French barber-surgeon, Ambroise Paré, to use a different treatment. During the Italian war of 1536–1538, Paré ran out of oil and instead used a balm of egg yolk, rose oil and turpentine [20]. He observed that the outcomes differed substantially between the two groups: those treated with the hot oil were feverish and in 'great pain and swelling about the edges of their wounds', whereas those given the balm were resting comfortably [21]. Further trials of the balm convinced Paré that gunshot wounds were not poisoned and should not be cauterised [20].

The comparison of groups also helped promote a technique for the prevention of smallpox. In the 1700s smallpox was a leading cause of death, with many of those who survived suffering disfigurement and blindness [22]. The available preventive measure was to infect children with puss or scab material from smallpox victims, a process known as variolation. Despite reports that it was beneficial [23], there was widespread concern that variolation might carry a greater risk of dying than allowing people to contract the disease naturally. James Jurin evaluated this in the 1720s, by collecting data on death rates in three groups: those who were diagnosed with smallpox, those at risk of contracting smallpox and those who had been variolated [22, 23]. The results appeared convincing with death rates of 16.5% (diagnosed cases), 8.3% (at risk) and 2.0% (variolated) [23]. Preventing smallpox was a much safer practice than letting nature take its course.

Death following childbirth was a serious concern in the seventeenth to nineteenth centuries, causing epidemics 'of unimaginable proportions' [24]. A major cause of this mortality, puerperal fever (fever following childbirth), was investigated by Ignaz Semmelweis, a Hungarian doctor. In 1844 he compared the death rates among patients in two wards of a hospital in Vienna. He found that the death rates in a ward staffed by doctors was much higher (16%) than in the one run by midwives (2%) [25]. This, and other observations, led Semmelweis to conclude that the illness was transmitted by doctors coming directly from a post-mortem to help deliver a baby. He initiated a preventive measure, compulsory hand washing in a chloride of lime solution, which reduced the mortality in the doctors' ward to 3% [25]. His approach was not popular, because it implied that doctors transmitted disease, and Semmelweis's contract was not renewed. He was finally vindicated some 30 years later when Pasteur identified the bacterium, *Streptococcus pyogenes*, that caused puerperal fever [25].

These treatment evaluations utilised two different types of comparisons: contemporary controls and historical controls. Contemporary controls are patients who were seen at the same time as those getting the new treatment, but who received the conventional care. Historical controls are patients who had been treated previously in the same location (e.g. hospital). Jurin's comparisons of groups at risk of smallpox, and Semmelweis's comparison of puerperal fever in two wards, used contemporary controls. In contrast the comparison of puerperal fever before and after introducing handwashing, and Paré's comparison of treatments for gunshot wounds, used historical control groups.

The problem with both types of control groups is that there could be systematic differences between the patients in the different groups. Isaac Massey, a contemporary of Jurin, made this criticism of the work on smallpox, pointing out that those who could afford variolation may have been in better health than those in the comparison groups [22]. He concluded that what was needed was groups that were similar, they 'must and ought to be as near as may be on a Par' [22].

COMPARING SIMILAR GROUPS

When groups are similar at baseline, it is more likely that any differences in subsequent outcomes will be due to the differences in the effects of the treatments. The idea of comparing like with like was proposed in the fourteenth century by the poet Francisco Petrarch, who suggested using similar groups of patients to compare the then current treatments with simply letting nature take its course [26].

One way to create similar groups is to recruit a number of patients who are all alike, then give them different treatments. The testing of potential treatments for scurvy is a widely cited example of the benefit of using similar groups. Scurvy is a debilitating and sometimes fatal disease, which afflicted sailors on long-distance sea voyages from the fifteenth to the nineteenth centuries [27, 28]. By the late 1500s, the benefits of consuming oranges and lemons were well known by Dutch sailors [27], but many English expeditions continued to suffer serious loss of life through scurvy [28]. The issue was still unresolved in 1747 when James Lind, a Royal Navy surgeon, carried out a classic study to assess the effects of six common treatments. He identified 12 sailors with scurvy who were 'as similar as I could have them', and tested each of the treatments on groups of 2 men (each pair to receive either: oil of vitriol, vinegar, sea water, cider, oranges and lemons, or a herbal paste) [29]. After 14 days Lind observed 'the most sudden and visible good effects were perceived from the use of oranges and lemons'. These findings were not widely accepted, and even Lind had doubts about them [29, 30], but the method used reflects an advance in thinking about ways to test treatments. Lind is rightly celebrated for his comparison of like with like in the evaluation of treatments. (In his 'Treatise of the Scurvy' Lind does not make any clear recommendations for the treatment of the disease, possibly because he believed that scurvy was not due to poor diet, but was a result of faulty digestion exacerbated by wet weather [29, 30].)

Another study in the eighteenth century used similar groups to assess whether the adverse effects of variolation (to prevent smallpox) could be ameliorated by pretreatment with a compound of mercury. At that time about 1 out of 50 patients vaccinated against smallpox died following the procedure [31]. In 1767 William Watson recruited 31 children who were similar in age, gender and diet [32]. These were divided into three groups, which received either the mercury mixture, a mild senna laxative or no treatment. No clear difference was found between the groups, using an objective measure of assessment (the number of pock marks caused by the variolation). Watson concluded that variolation against smallpox was effective with or without pretreatment with mercury or a mild laxative [32].

CASTING LOTS AND TREATMENT ALLOCATION

Comparing similar groups of patients was an important step forward in the evaluation of treatments, but it leaves open the possibility that the groups may have differed on important factors that were not measured. Further, a subconscious bias in the doctor allocating patients to treatments could influence the way individuals were assigned to groups (e.g. the slightly sicker ones might be preferentially assigned to one group). An alternative approach, which prevents this bias, is to allocate individuals to treatments in a truly random way, so that the final groups will be balanced on all factors, whether measured or not.

The idea that some form of randomisation should be used to allocate patients to treatment groups was proposed in the 1640s. Joan Baptista van Helmont, a Flemish chemist, alchemist and physician, recommended this method to evaluate the effectiveness of bloodletting [33]. He suggested dividing up to 500 patients into 2 groups, then casting lots (equivalent to tossing a coin) to decide which group would be given the conventional therapy (bloodletting) and which would receive van Helmont's own treatment. A notable feature of the trial design is that the outcome would be decided by the number of funerals that occurred in the two groups. The experiment was not carried out. (The proposed use of an objective outcome measure such as this is unusual for its time.)

One method of randomised allocation was used in 1848 by Thomas Graham Balfour to investigate whether homeopathic belladonna could prevent scarlet fever. Balfour identified 151 boys who had not had the disease, and 'divided them into two sections, taking them alternately from the list, to prevent the imputation of selection' [34]. Balfour recognised that if he had to decide which boys were allocated to each group, his choices might be biased. (Alternate selection from a list is essentially a method of randomisation, as the factors which are related to dying from scarlet fever, will be randomly scattered throughout the list.) The study showed that exactly two children in each group developed scarlet fever, leading him to conclude that 'the numbers are too small to justify deductions as to the prophylactic power of belladonna' [34], a commendably careful interpretation of the findings.

Instead of alternate selection from a list, patients could be allocated to treatments by the date of their admission to hospital. This method was used by the Danish physician Johannes Fibiger in 1896–1897 [35] to evaluate the effectiveness of a serum treatment for diphtheria. Thus, patients admitted to hospital on one day received serum and those on the next day were untreated. The outcome was persuasive: only 8 of 239 patients in the serum group died, compared to 30 of the 245 controls.

The use of alternate allocation began to gain popularity in the first few decades of the twentieth century because it prevented bias in the assignment of patients to treatments. These research studies were conducted in both the United States and the UK, with patients being randomised by the order of their attendance at a healthcare facility [36–39]. These trials signalled the growing recognition of the importance of achieving comparable groups.

RANDOM NUMBERS FOR TREATMENT ALLOCATION

A landmark series of three trials, conducted under the auspices of the UK Medical Research Council, used random numbers to allocate patients to treatments. This methodological advance was proposed by the medical statistician Professor (later Sir) Austin Bradford Hill [40]. It was first used in a large field trial that assessed the effectiveness of a vaccine for whooping cough [41]. Although this study began in 1944, it was not published until 1951. The second trial, of streptomycin for pulmonary tuberculosis, became the most highly acclaimed study in the history of treatment evaluation. It began in 1946, but was the first to be published, in 1948 [42]. The third trial involved a large-scale field trial of an antihistaminic drug (thonzylamine) for the prevention of the common cold [43].

As well as being published first, the streptomycin trial provided a major advance in the treatment of a feared disease, tuberculosis: it reduced the fatality rate at six months from 27% to 7% and also reduced the severity of disease among survivors. An editorial that accompanied the paper identified the advantage of individual randomisation over alternate allocation: it prevented a patient being included or rejected, based on whether the next treatment was to be antibiotic or control [44]. For example, if the doctor thought that the drug would not be effective in seriously ill patients, they might not be included in the study if they were scheduled to receive the active treatment. This would only need to happen a few times to bias the results of the study.

In addition to the use of random numbers to allocate patients to treatments, these three trials stand out for two other reasons. Patients were recruited from multiple centres to provide sufficient participants to be able to draw firm conclusions. The researchers also made considerable efforts to ensure that the participants, and the clinicians measuring the outcomes, were unaware of which treatment the patients received. This prevented bias in the reporting of symptoms by participants, and by those recording the outcomes: in modern terminology, it was double blind.

The landmark streptomycin trial in tuberculosis was followed by another study on pulmonary tuberculosis, published two years later [45]. It compared three treatments: streptomycin, another drug, para-amino-salicylic acid (PAS), and a combination of these two drugs. The same methodology was used as in the first streptomycin trial. The combination therapy had the best outcome, with streptomycin coming second. More importantly the combined treatment led to a much lower frequency of bacterial resistance to streptomycin. This study has been credited with leading to the maxim 'never treat active tuberculosis with a single agent', which is now the standard for managing this disease [46]. The clinical benefits apart, this set of four rigorous studies supported by the Medical Research Council inaugurated the era of high quality clinical trials.

THE NEED FOR BLINDING

A major concern of several trials in the middle of the twentieth century was to ensure that the patients and clinical observers were unaware of how treatments were allocated [39, 41, 43]. This would prevent knowledge of who received which treatment from influencing the outcome of the study. The idea was not new; it featured in studies to evaluate a treatment called animal magnetism. This treatment was championed in the late 1700s by Franz Anton Mesmer, who believed he could impart magnetic energy and thereby cure a wide range of illnesses [47]. Mesmer achieved great fame, and a lucrative medical practice in Paris. This popularity was of such concern to other doctors, and to the government, that they persuaded Louis XVI to establish a Royal Commission to evaluate the claims of cures and dramatic effects [47, 48]. The Commission conducted a series of studies in which participants either thought they were being magnetised (when they were not), or thought they were not subjected to magnetism (when they were). The findings were convincing. Participants only reported benefits when they (falsely) believed they were being treated: 'the imagination is the real cause of the effects attributed to magnetism' [47]. Following publication of the Commission's report, Mesmer was ridiculed, and animal magnetism was abandoned in France.

A more recent example of the importance of blinding is the evaluation of a surgical technique, internal-mammary artery-ligation, for the relief of angina symptoms. Several reports in the 1950s had claimed that the operation provided considerable relief of symptoms [49, 50]. This prompted two groups of researchers to carry out controlled trials to evaluate the effectiveness of the surgery. Patients were randomly allocated to have artery ligation, or to a control group which received a sham operation involving only a skin incision. The patients, and the cardiologists who evaluated the outcomes, were blind to treatment group. The ligation operation provided no benefit, as most patients in both the treatment group and in the control group reported significant improvement in symptoms [49, 50]. The authors concluded that these claims were most likely a psychological response to undergoing surgery.

The response to a sham treatment is known as a placebo effect. Understanding of the psychological and physiological factors underlying the placebo response has advanced greatly in recent years [51, 52]. A consistent finding is that patients who have high expectations of their treatment usually experience improvements in symptoms. If patients were aware of their treatment allocation, only those in the active group would have the high expectations. Concealment of treatment allocation could prevent this bias from creating difference between the groups.

CONCLUSION

Obtaining evidence on treatment effectiveness is a challenging business. As Passamani remarked in 1991, 'The history of medicine is richly endowed with therapies that were widely used and then shown to be ineffective or frankly toxic' [53]. A similar view was expressed by the celebrated American physician, Oliver Wendell Holmes in 1860, 'if the whole materia medica, as now used, could be sunk to the bottom of the sea, it would be all the better for mankind – and all the worse for the fishes' [54]. These may seem somewhat jaundiced views, but they reflect the large proportion of ineffective and possibly harmful treatments that were once used. Even in the early years of the twentieth century many ineffective treatments were widely used [55], and some treatments of little value continue to be used today [56]. Concern about this has led to a recent international campaign, 'Choosing Wisely', to reduce the use of ineffective or harmful treatments [57].

This chapter has presented examples of different approaches used to identify potentially effective treatments. Reliance on theories of disease processes is often unreliable and can result in harmful treatments being used. Careful observation of treatment outcomes in a series of patients can, if the benefits are immediate and substantial, identify effective treatments. Comparisons of groups of patients given different treatments are often more insightful, but are vulnerable to the criticism that the groups might not be similar at baseline. As the eminent French physician P C A Louis pointed out in 1834, 'it is necessary to account for differences of age, sex, temperament, physical condition, natural history of the disease' [58]. The use of groups constructed to be similar on some factors at baseline is a definite improvement, but leaves open the question that they differ on other (unmeasured) factors. Allocation of individual patients to treatments using random numbers overcomes two problems: clinician bias in assigning patients to groups, and differences in unmeasured factors.

The sequence of methods presented in this chapter could be taken to imply that there was a steady progression to increased robustness of study design. However, as the dates for the individual studies show, there is little evidence for continuous improvement in methods: rather there was substantial overlap in the use of these methods. The major advances in trial methodology occurred in studies conducted in the middle of the twentieth century. They used three techniques that are now hallmarks of high quality trials: randomisation, blinding of the investigators and patients to the randomisation process, and objective outcome measures.

In summary, this chapter has reviewed the development of methods to evaluate treatments up to the middle of the twentieth century. It has highlighted pitfalls of many of the earlier methods and concluded with an outline of the advantages of the double blind randomised controlled trial. This method is now used around the world to identify the benefits of treatments. Medicine now has the tools to ensure that only effective treatments are used. The next chapter explores whether the benefits of the randomised controlled trial have been realised.

REFERENCES

1. Porter, R. (1999). *The Greatest Benefit to Mankind*. London: Harpers Collins.
2. Cantu, J.Q. (1965). Benjamin Franklin's medical imprints. *Bull. Med. Libr. Assoc.* 53: 71–79.
3. Bhatt, A. (2010). Evolution of clinical research: a history before and beyond Lames Lind. *Perspect. Clin. Res.* 1: 6–10.
4. Ackerknecht, E.H. (1982). *A Short History of Medicine*. Baltimore: Johns Hopkins University Press.
5. DePalma, R.G., Hayes, V.W., and Zacharski, L.R. (2007). Bloodletting: past and present. *J. Am. Coll. Surg.* 205: 132–144.
6. Risse, G.B. (1979). Renaissance of bloodletting – chapter in modern therapeutics. *J. Hist. Med. Allied Sci.* 34: 3–22.
7. Stokes, W. (1865). The address in medicine. *BMJ* ii: 133–142.
8. Biggio, J.R. Jr. (2013). Bed rest in pregnancy: time to put the issue to rest. *Obstet. Gynecol.* 121: 1158–1160.
9. Sprague, A.E. (2004). The evolution of bed rest as a clinical intervention. *J. Obstet. Gynecol. Neonatal. Nurs.* 33: 542–549.

10. Bigelow, C. and Stone, J. (2011). Bed rest in pregnancy. *Mt Sinai J. Med.* 78: 291–302.
11. McCall, C.A., Grimes, D.A., and Lyerly, A.D. (2013). 'Therapeutic' bed rest in pregnancy: unethical and unsupported by data. *Obstet. Gynecol.* 121: 1305–1308.
12. Brower, R.G. (2009). Consequences of bed rest. *Crit. Care Med.* 37: S422–S428.
13. Jack, D.B. (1997). One hundred years of aspirin. *Lancet* 350: 437–439.
14. Montinari, M.R., Minelli, S., and De Caterina, R. (2019). The first 3500years of aspirin history from its roots – a concise summary. *Vasc. Pharmacol.* 113: 1–8.
15. Vane, J.R., Flower, R.J., and Botting, R.M. (1990). History of aspirin and its mechanism of action. *Stroke* 21: IV12–IV23.
16. Rosenfeld, L. (2002). Insulin: discovery and controversy. *Clin. Chem.* 48: 2270–2288.
17. Banting, F.G. (1926). An address on diabetes and insulin: being the Nobel lecture delivered at Stockholm on September 15th, 1925. *CMAJ* 16: 221–232.
18. Banting, F.G., Best, C.H., Collip, J.B. et al. (1922). Pancreatic extracts in the treatment of diabetes mellitus. *CMAJ* 12: 141–146.
19. Karamitsos, D.T. (2011). The story of insulin discovery. *Diabetes Res. Clin. Pract.* 93 (Suppl 1): S2–S8.
20. Wangensteen, O.H., Wangensteen, S.D., and Klinger, C.F. (1972). Wound management of Ambroise pare and Dominique Larrey, great French military surgeons of the 16th and 19th centuries. *Bull. Hist. Med.* 46: 207–234.
21. Drucker, C.B. (2008). Ambroise pare and the birth of the gentle art of surgery. *Yale J. Biol. Med.* 81: 199–202.
22. Huth, E. (2006). Quantitative evidence for judgments on the efficacy of inoculation for the prevention of smallpox: England and New England in the 1700s. *J. R. Soc. Med.* 99: 262–266.
23. Bird, A. (2019). James Jurin and the avoidance of bias in collecting and assessing evidence on the effects of variolation. *J. R. Soc. Med.* 112: 119–123.

24. Charles, D. and Larsen, B. (1986). Streptococcal puerperal sepsis and obstetric infections: a historical perspective. *Rev. Infect. Dis.* 8: 411–422.

25. Adriaanse, A.H., Pel, M., and Bleker, O.P. (2000). Semmelweis: the combat against puerperal fever. *Eur. J. Obstet. Gynecol. Reprod. Biol.* 90: 153–158.

26. Chalmers, I., Dukan, E., Podolsky, S. et al. (2012). The advent of fair treatment allocation schedules in clinical trials during the 19th and early 20th centuries. *J. R. Soc. Med.* 105: 221–227.

27. Burnby, J. and Bierman, A. (1996). The incidence of scurvy at sea and its treatment. *Rev. Hist. Pharm.* 44: 339–346.

28. Baron, J.H. (2009). Sailors' scurvy before and after James Lind – a reassessment. *Nutr. Rev.* 67: 315–332.

29. Milne, I. (2012). Who was James Lind, and what exactly did he achieve. *J. R. Soc. Med.* 105: 503–508.

30. Bartholomew, M. (2002). James Lind's treatise of the scurvy (1753). *Postgrad. Med. J.* 78: 695–696.

31. Boylston, A.W. (2002). Clinical investigation of smallpox in 1767. *N. Engl. J. Med.* 346: 1326–1328.

32. Boylston, A. (2014). William Watson's use of controlled clinical experiments in 1767. *J. R. Soc. Med.* 107: 246–248.

33. Donaldson, I.M. (2016). Van Helmont's proposal for a randomised comparison of treating fevers with or without bloodletting and purging. *J. R. Coll. Physicians Edinb.* 46: 206–213.

34. Chalmers, I. and Toth, B. (2009). Nineteenth-century controlled trials to test whether belladonna prevents scarlet fever. *J. R. Soc. Med.* 102: 549–550.

35. Hrobjartsson, A., Gotzsche, P.C., and Gluud, C. (1998). The controlled clinical trial turns 100 years: Fibiger's trial of serum treatment of diphtheria. *BMJ* 317: 1243–1245.

36. Podolsky, S.H. (2009). Jesse Bullowa, specific treatment for pneumonia, and the development of the controlled clinical trial. *J. R. Soc. Med.* 102: 203–207.

37. MRC (1934). The serum treatment of lobar pneumonia: a report of the therapeutic trials Committee of the Medical Research Council. *BMJ* 1: 241–245.

38. Lorriman, G. and Martin, W.J. (1950). Trial of antistin in the common cold. *BMJ* 2: 430–431.

39. MRC (2004). Clinical trial of patulin in the common cold. 1944. *Int. J. Epidemiol.* 33: 243–246.

40. Hill, A.B. (1990). Suspended judgment. Memories of the British streptomycin trial in tuberculosis. The first randomized clinical trial. *Control. Clin. Trials* 11: 77–79.

41. MRC (1951). Prevention of whooping-cough by vaccination; a Medical Research Council investigation. *BMJ* 1: 1463–1471.

42. MRC (1948). Streptomycin treatment of pulmonary tuberculosis. *BMJ* 2: 769–782.

43. MRC (1950). Clinical trials of antihistaminic drugs in the prevention and treatment of the common cold; report by a special committee of the Medical Research Council. *BMJ* 2: 425–429.

44. Editorial (1948). The controlled therapeutic trial. *BMJ* 2: 791–792.

45. MRC (1950). Treatment of pulmonary tuberculosis with streptomycin and Para-aminosalicylic acid; a Medical Research Council investigation. *BMJ* 2: 1073–1085.

46. Murray, J.F., Schraufnagel, D.E., and Hopewell, P.C. (2015). Treatment of tuberculosis. A historical perspective. *Ann. Am. Thorac. Soc.* 12: 1749–1759.

47. Lanska, D.J. and Lanska, J.T. (2007). Franz Anton Mesmer and the rise and fall of animal magnetism: dramatic cures, controversy, and ultimately a triumph for the scientific method. In: *Brain, Mind and Medicine: Essays in Eighteenth-Century Neuroscience* (eds. H. Whitaker, C.U.M. Smith and S. Finger), 301–320. New York: Springer https://doi.org/10.1007/978-0-387-70967-3.

48. Donaldson, I.M. (2005). Mesmer's 1780 proposal for a controlled trial to test his method of treatment using "animal magnetism". *J. R. Soc. Med.* 98: 572–575.

49. Dimond, E.G., Kittle, C.F., and Crockett, J.E. (1960). Comparison of internal mammary artery ligation and sham operation for angina pectoris. *Am. J. Cardiol.* 5: 483–486.

50. Cobb, L.A., Thomas, G.I., Dillard, D.H. et al. (1959). An evaluation of internal-mammary-artery ligation by a double-blind technic. *N. Engl. J. Med.* 260: 1115–1118.

51. Enck, P., Bingel, U., Schedlowski, M. et al. (2013). The placebo response in medicine: minimize, maximize or personalize? *Nat. Rev. Drug Discov.* 12: 191–204.

52. Horing, B., Weimer, K., Muth, E.R. et al. (2014). Prediction of placebo responses: a systematic review of the literature. *Front. Psychol.* https://doi.org/10.3389/fpsyg.2014.01079.

53. Passamani, E. (1991). Clinical trials – are they ethical? *N. Engl. J. Med.* 324: 1589–1592.

54. Schimmel, E.M. (1963). The physician as pathogen. *J. Chronic Dis.* 16: 1–4.

55. Beeson, P.B. (1980). Changes in medical therapy during the past half century. *Medicine* 59: 79–99.

56. Mafi, J.N. and Parchman, M. (2018). Low-value care: an intractable global problem with no quick fix. *BMJ Qual. Saf.* 27: 333–336.

57. Levinson, W., Kallewaard, M., Bhatia, R.S. et al. (2015). 'Choosing Wisely': a growing international campaign. *BMJ Qual. Saf.* 24: 167–174.

58. Best, M. and Neuhauser, D. (2005). Pierre Charles Alexandre Louis: master of the spirit of mathematical clinical science. *Qual. Saf. Health Care* 14: 462–464.

CHAPTER 2

Sources of Bias in Randomised Controlled Trials

The great strength of randomised controlled trials is that they provide a fair comparison of treatments. However flaws in the design and conduct of clinical trials can hamper the ability to make fair comparisons. This chapter explores the nature and frequency of these problems. It uses the findings from meta-research studies that explore the quality of the methodology of large series of clinical trials, to identify the extent of these deficiencies [1, 2].

In essence, clinical trials are conducted in three stages. First, patients are allocated to receive the new treatment or the conventional one (or placebo). Then they are followed up over time to allow the effects of the treatment to occur. Finally the health status of the patients is assessed to show whether the new treatment has a better outcome than the comparator.

Evidence in Medicine: The Common Flaws, Why They Occur and How to Prevent Them, First Edition. Iain K Crombie.
© 2021 John Wiley & Sons Ltd. Published 2021 by John Wiley & Sons Ltd.

This chapter explores the types of flaws that occur at these three stages. The main concern is with the risk of bias. Bias occurs when the findings of a clinical trial do not provide a fair assessment of the true benefit of the new treatment. Poor quality of the study methods can increase the risk of bias. This chapter investigates the sources of bias and the impact these have on estimates of treatment effect.

METHOD OF TREATMENT ALLOCATION

In clinical trials patients are assigned to different treatment groups using a sequence of random numbers. The process of randomisation produces two groups that, on average, are similar at baseline on factors such as severity and duration of disease. When the groups are similar at baseline, any differences between them at follow-up will be due to the effect of the treatment. Deficiencies in the method of randomisation could cause imbalances at baseline, resulting in differences in outcomes between the groups that are unrelated to treatment. This section identifies the problems that frequently occur with treatment allocation.

Generation of the Random Assignment

Meta-research studies have shown that the randomisation process is often flawed. For many trials the method is not described, is poorly described, or is well described but clearly inadequate [3–5]. An evaluation of 2 groups of trials, comprising 1,376 and 984 studies, found that 39.6% and 52.2% had flawed or poorly reported methods for generating the randomisation sequence [6].

The recommended method of randomising patients is by computer-generated random numbers. Other techniques, such as allocation by day of admission to hospital or by even or odd dates of birth, have been used, but are thought to be unreliable. Careful reviews of large series of trials have shown that poor quality and inadequately described methods of generating the randomisation sequence commonly exaggerate the apparent benefit of treatment [4, 7].

Importance of Concealed Allocation

The assignment of patients to treatment should correspond exactly to the randomisation sequence. However the process could be distorted, if the clinician recruiting the patient knew in advance which treatment the next patient would be given. For example, concerns about possible side effects might lead a clinician to decide not to recruit more severely ill patients if they were to be randomised to receive the new treatment. Thus fewer severely ill patients would be allocated to the active treatment. The resulting differences between the groups at baseline would bias the estimate of treatment benefit.

The solution is to ensure those involved in the trial have no access to the randomisation sequence, a process called allocation concealment. To achieve this, the randomisation is commonly handled by a remote site, such as a clinical trials unit, which could, for example, provide the treatments in separate containers labelled A or B. The methods used to conceal treatment allocation should be clearly described in the trial report, to give reassurance that bias is unlikely to have occurred.

Overviews of trials have shown that inadequate or poorly reported methods of allocation concealment are common. A major review of over 20,000 trials found that allocation concealment was adequate in only 35% of trials [5]. Other overviews in different clinical specialties found that the process was adequately described in 53% of neurological trials [8], 43% of surgical trials [3] and 27% of trials in multiple sclerosis [9]. An extreme example comes from the field of oral health in which only 15% of trials had low risk of bias for allocation concealment [10]. These studies suggest that as many as two third of trials are at risk of producing biased estimates of treatment.

Evidence that the Randomisation Process Is Subverted

Randomisation will usually produce two treatment groups with similar sample sizes, but only rarely will they have identical numbers of patients. A review found that many more trials had groups with identical sample sizes than could occur by chance [11]. The conclusion is that someone may have modified the randomisation sequence to prevent disparity in the size of the two groups, an action described as 'forcing cosmetic credibility' [11].

Randomisation should also result in the two groups being similar at baseline on characteristics such as age and clinical signs and symptoms. Small differences between groups commonly occur, but many trials have much more marked imbalances between groups than would be expected by chance. This has been documented for participant age [12] and for important clinical predictors of outcome [13]. These imbalances suggest that the randomisation sequence has been altered, with the likely consequence that the estimates of treatment effect will be biased.

A few studies have explored whether researchers admit to deciphering the randomisation sequence. Schulz and colleagues found that many clinicians try to decode the sequence [14]. Paludan-Muller and colleagues [15] reviewed surveys of the reasons why clinicians do this. The most common reasons were that a doctor had a preference for a treatment for a particular patient, or had a desire to show that the new treatment was effective. Some researchers admitted to distorting the randomisation sequence by entering two or more patients at the same time, so that a particular patient could be allocated to a preferred treatment [15]. In some trials the treatment allocation codes are delivered in sealed envelopes [16], enabling some clinicians to subvert the randomisation by opening the envelopes before entering the patients [15]. Whatever the method of manipulation, deviations from random allocation could lead to bias.

Does Integrity of Allocation Concealment Matter?

A seminal paper by Schulz and colleagues in 1995 showed that studies that reported inadequate concealment treatment allocation exaggerate the estimates of treatment benefit [17]. The initial overview evaluated 250 trials of interventions in pregnancy and childbirth. Since then this finding has been replicated and extended by two overview studies covering thousands of trials across all areas of medicine [7, 18]. Their finding is that poor or inadequately described methods of allocation concealment lead to exaggerated treatment effects.

PROBLEMS IN MEASURING THE OUTCOME

The effectiveness of a treatment is assessed by comparing the health status of those in the intervention and control groups at the end of the trial. In many clinical settings the effect of treatment could be measured by several different outcomes. For example, in cancer trials possible outcomes would include the average survival time, disease-free survival or quality of life. Commonly, one outcome measure is designated the primary outcome, with the other outcomes being termed secondary measures. (This is to prevent researchers from analysing many different outcomes, then highlighting the one which looks best.) Selecting the primary outcome involves difficult choices, but it greatly simplifies the interpretation of the results.

Switching Primary Outcomes

Before recruiting patients, many trials report their detailed methods in an international trial register. Several international registers have been established (e.g. ClinicalTrials.gov and the ISRCTN registry) [19, 20]. Many researchers also publish their study protocols in a medical journal. These sources allow other researchers to compare the outcome measures that were initially specified with those that are presented in the publication of the trial results. A review of outcome reporting in high quality neurology journals found that in 180 trials, 21% of the specified primary outcomes had been omitted, 6% of primary outcomes were demoted to secondary outcomes and 34% of trials added previously unmentioned primary outcomes [21]. A similar pattern was seen in trials published in haematology journals where 40% of primary outcomes had been omitted, 25% of primary outcomes were demoted and many new outcomes were added [22]. The evidence is clear that in trials across the medical specialties, primary outcomes are frequently changed [23–26].

Outcomes may be changed for good reasons, such as replacing a difficult to measure outcome with a more amenable one. But there may be other motives. Several studies have shown that the effect of substituting outcomes favours the publication of positive findings

[21, 26]; that is when a non-significant primary outcome is demoted and a significant secondary one is promoted to primary outcome. Compared to trials with unchanged outcomes, those with substituted outcomes report an increased effect size [27].

One study explored why authors had omitted or changed outcomes [28]; often this was because the researchers thought that a non-significant result was not interesting. A review of such studies found that a preference for positive finding, and a poor or flexible research design, were the reasons most commonly mentioned for switching outcomes [29]. It seems likely that outcomes are sometimes changed based on the findings from an initial analysis.

Blinding of Outcome Assessment

A long-standing feature of trials is that the patient, and the person who measures patient status (the outcome) at the end of the trial, should be unaware of (blinded to) the treatment the participants received. This ensures that knowledge of treatment group does not influence the way the outcome is measured.

In many trials the method of blinding outcome assessment is poor. An evaluation of 20,920 trials included in Cochrane systematic reviews found that 31% of trials had unclear risk of blinding of participants and a further 33% were at high risk of bias [5]. For outcome assessment, 25% were at unclear risk of and 23% were at high risk of bias [5].

Another concern is whether blinding is compromised. This can happen when an intervention is sufficiently different from the control (e.g. by taste) that the patient identifies which treatment they have been given, and reveals this to the outcome assessor [30]. Few studies report whether they have assessed the risk that unblinding has occurred [31]. However one study that contacted the authors of published trials found that 43% has assessed this risk without reporting it, and that in 11% of studies it was likely that blinding had been compromised [30].

The impact of poor quality blinding on estimates of treatment effect is unclear, as review studies give conflicting results. Two overview studies found that poor blinding was associated with an increased effect size compared to well-blinded trials [7, 32]. Another study found that this bias only occurred for subjective outcome measures [2], and a fourth reported an inconsistent effect [18]. The most recent, and largest, study concluded that there was no effect of blinding [33].

Reporting of Adverse Events

A basic principle of pharmacology is that 'all drugs have beneficial and harmful effects' [34], with the value of the drug depending on the benefit: harm ratio. Establishing where the balance lies can be difficult because the harms are frequently under-reported in published clinical trials [35, 36]. One study found that 43% of adverse events recorded in trial registries were not reported in the published study [37]. A review of such studies concluded that, on average, some 64% of harms were not reported [38]. The benefit: harm ratio may often be biased because of the under-reporting of harms [39].

FOLLOW-UP AND MISSING OUTCOMES

In a trial, patients are followed up for a defined period to determine the effect of treatment. During this time period some patients can withdraw from the study, and contact can be lost with others, so that the outcome is often not measured on all patients. A rule of thumb for losses to follow-up is that <5% loss is unlikely to cause bias and that >20% loss is serious, with those between 5% and 20% being potentially problematic [40, 41].

Extent of Loss to Follow-up

Loss to follow-up occurs in almost all clinical trials, although reporting of this is often incomplete. One problem is that some published papers give no information about loss to follow-up. A study of trials in five leading journals found that 13% failed to report whether or not loss to follow-up had occurred [42]. Other studies have found that the lack of an explicit statement about missing data occurred in 6.5% [43] and 26% [44] of published papers.

Trials that report the extent of loss to follow-up vary greatly in the proportion of participants affected. Among 77 trials published in leading medical journals in 2013, 95% reported some missing outcome data: although the median loss was 9%, the highest reported was 70% [45]. Similarly in trials funded by a Health Technology Assessment programme, the median loss was 11%, but this ranged from 0% to 77% in individual studies [46].

In many trials loss follow-up exceeds the notional threshold of 20% for serious loss. The extent of this may vary across specialties. Among trials in palliative care it was 23% [47], slightly higher in osteoarthritis (26%) [44] and 39% in rheumatoid arthritis [48]. Among obesity trials 74% reported losses >20% [49].

Care is needed in the interpretation of the loss to follow-up rates. In a study of 21 trials, the data reported to the US Food and Drugs Administration showed markedly higher median loss to follow-up (13%), than that in the corresponding published papers (0.3%) [50]. The authors of this study concluded that the 'published rates consistently seem to be inadequate representations of the completeness and quality of follow-up'.

Characteristics of Patients Lost

The type of patient lost to follow-up is possibly more important than the number lost. If more seriously ill patients are lost, and this loss happens to a greater extent in one of the treatment groups, then substantial bias can occur. Thus when loss to follow-up occurs, trials need to report not just the magnitude of loss, but the number and characteristics of the patients lost from each of the treatment arms.

Trials that report the overall loss to follow-up often do not give the data separately for intervention and control groups. One study of trials in leading medical journals found that 20% did not report the numbers missing in the treatment and control groups separately [42]. However a more recent study found that leading journals had improved, with only 3% of trials failing to report this information [45]. Another study of trials in palliative care found that 13% did not report the numbers lost to follow-up in both treatment arms [51]. In these studies it is not clear whether treatment effects will be biased by differential loss to follow-up.

Reporting of the types of patients lost to follow-up is often poor. In one review, 91% of trials did not compare the characteristics of those lost to follow-up with those successfully followed up [43]. Among 108 trials in palliative care, none compared the intervention and control groups for the baseline characteristics of those with missing outcome data [47]. Thus it is often not possible to assess whether those lost to follow-up in the intervention group differ from those lost in the control group.

Bias from Loss to Follow-up

The impact of loss to follow-up is difficult to predict. A review found that loss to follow-up was sometimes higher in the treatment group and sometimes in the comparator [47]. Possibly the effect of loss to follow-up depends on the specific trial characteristics, such as the illness being treated or the acceptability of the treatment to patients. Whatever the explanation, concern remains that some trials may be biased due to patient attrition.

MISSING OUTCOME DATA AND INTENTION TO TREAT

A difficult issue for the analysis of a trial is how to cope with those who are lost to follow-up. The accepted approach to this problem is termed 'intention to treat'. This holds that all patients should be analysed in the groups to which they were randomised, no matter what subsequently happened to them. Intention to treat is regarded as 'a key defence against bias' in clinical trials [52].

A popular technique to handle missing data is complete case analysis, which restricts the analysis to those successfully followed up. This approach was used in 26% of trials on musculoskeletal disorders [53], in 45%–54% of studies in general medicine [45, 54] and in 60% of trials in palliative care [51]. Despite its popularity, complete case analysis clearly contravenes the principle of intention to treat, effectively losing the benefit of randomisation. This method is likely to introduce bias, because the number and types of patients lost to follow-up are unlikely to be the same in the intervention and control groups [55].

Methods of Imputation

Instead of ignoring the problem, as complete case analysis does, a better approach is to use a method to estimate what the missing value might be. This is termed imputation. The simplest form of imputation is last observation carried forward. If trials measure the outcome at more than one time point, the most recent observation is used in the analysis; if there are no intermediate measures the baseline measurement is used. This method is often used in trials [45, 48], but it has been heavily criticised because it is likely to lead to biased estimates of treatment effects [55–57]. As disease severity often changes over time, with relapses or remissions, early values can be poor predictors of the final outcome.

Multiple imputation is a more sophisticated approach to estimate the missing outcome data. It uses statistical modelling to derive estimates of the missing data based on the available data (imputation). The modelling includes the variables that would normally be used in the final analysis, such as the stratification variables (e.g. centre, gender), treatment group and potential confounders (e.g. initial disease severity, other medical conditions). It can also include other variables (auxiliary variables) that might be available [58, 59]. The idea is that patient characteristics, both medical and demographic, could predict the final outcome. The modelling process is repeated many times to produce an average result (hence multiple imputation).

Multiple imputation makes an assumption about the nature of the missingness of the data. Termed 'missing at random', the assumption is that the missing outcomes can be predicted from the other data in the study [60]. It is recommended that sensitivity analysis should be used to explore the effect of assumptions about the missing data [59]. Although not a perfect solution, multiple imputation is better than other methods of dealing with missing data (such as complete case analysis or last observation carried forward) [58].

Modified Intention to Treat

The term modified intention to treat (mITT) is commonly used to describe the analysis of trial data [61, 62]. It has no formal definition [63], but usually involves the deliberate exclusion of some participants from the analysis at some time after randomisation. Patients can be excluded for several reasons: the results of the baseline assessment; results of a post-baseline assessment; the amount of treatment received; or failure to obtain the outcome measures [63]. Individual trials could employ one or more of these reasons to exclude patients. The impact of mITT on estimates of treatment benefit varies: one review found that, compared to intention to treat (ITT) analyses, the modified method inflated treatment effects [64], whereas another study found no difference between ITT and mITT [65]. The practice of excluding patients after randomisation has been widely criticised because of its potential to introduce bias [62, 66, 67].

OTHER METHODOLOGICAL CONCERNS

Unregistered Trials and Bias

Trial registration 'was introduced in an effort to reduce publication bias and raise the quality of clinical research' [68]. Although registration is strongly recommended, a recent study showed that only 53% of trials had had done so [69]. An analysis of over 1,100 trials explored the factors associated with registration. Compared to registered studies, trials that are unregistered are more likely to be of lower methodological quality. For example, they are less likely to have a defined primary outcome (48% vs 88%), more likely to have not reported or inadequate allocation concealment (76% vs 55%), less likely to report whether or not blinded (32% vs 15%), and more likely not to report details of attrition (67% vs 29%) [70]. When adjusted for methodological weaknesses, the unregistered trials had a modest increase in the average effect size compared to the registered studies. Another study evaluated 322 trials, and also showed a similar modest effect on treatment effect estimates [71]. Unregistered trials may give biased estimates of treatment effect.

Small Studies

Small trials often give misleading estimates of treatment benefit. Several review studies, each of which examined hundreds of trials, have shown that, on average, small trials report greater effect sizes than larger ones [72–74]. Two explanations have been suggested for this finding: small studies with negative findings may be less likely to be published, and small studies may be of poorer methodological quality and more prone to bias [73]. Most likely both factors contribute to the bias.

A related phenomenon is that unusually large treatment effects are most commonly reported by small trials [75]. These often occur in the first trial of a new treatment, with subsequent trials showing much smaller effects [76–78]. A possible explanation for this is that small studies are much more likely to be influenced by the play of chance [79]. A few more events (e.g. deaths) in one treatment group, or a few less in the other, can have a large effect on small studies. When averaged across many trials, chance effects cancel out, but for an individual study it can generate large, misleading effect sizes.

The fragility index is used to identify just how susceptible statistically significant results are to the play of chance [80]. It measures how many fewer events would have to occur to change a significant treatment effect to a non-significant one. Reviews have found that for many trials the index is one i.e. if one patient had a different outcome the finding would not be statistically significant [81, 82]. In general, the smaller the value of the index, the more fragile the study. Several reviews of trials have reported the median values of the index of 1, 2, 3 and 4 [82–84], indicating that, for half of the trials included in these reviews, a different outcome in a few patients would change the statistical significance. Other reviews have found slightly larger median fragility indices of 5 and 8 [80, 85].

Low Power

Small studies are often referred to as having low power. In medical research, statistical power refers to the chances (probability) that a study will detect a significant effect of treatment if one truly exists. A power of 80% is recommended, but few trials in medicine achieve this: in an overview of 136,000 trials only 9% of those published between 2010 and 2014 did so [86].

A consequence of low power is that spuriously significant results are more likely to occur [87]. Another problem is that, if there is a real benefit of treatment, small studies are unlikely to detect the benefit as being statistically significant. These apparently conflicting statements are true because chance is even-handed; it will make some interventions appear to have a larger effect size than they do in reality, and will sometimes make the effect seem smaller than it really is [79]. Inflated effect sizes are more likely to be significant and reduced ones less so. The result is that small trials have much more heterogeneous effect sizes than large ones [88].

To ensure that the trial has adequate power, researchers should carry out a formal sample size calculation (specifying the likely size of the treatment effect as well as the required power and an estimate of variance). The frequency of reporting sample size calculations is often low. For example, only 41% of low back pain trials [89] and 35% neurosurgical trials [90] reported this calculation. Even when the sample size calculation is reported, researchers often overestimate the possible benefit of the treatment and end up with sample sizes that are too small to detect a clinically realistic effect [89, 91].

Industry-Funded Trials

The research funded by drug companies 'produces innovative, life-saving medicines', but it also has a darker side [92]. A common finding is that trials funded by the pharmaceutical industry are more likely to report that the treatment was beneficial [93, 94]. One review study concluded that 'pharmaceutical company sponsorship is strongly associated with results that favour the sponsor's interests' [95]. Another author commented that 'big pharma is more concerned about commercial interests than patient harm' [96]. Editors of leading medical journals, and reviews by academic researchers, have heavily criticised the pharmaceutical industry for sponsoring trials whose results 'favour the sponsors' interests' [93, 97, 98]. As industry fund the majority of large international trials, and is particularly good at disseminating their findings [99], any bias in their studies could create serious problems for evidence. Many industry-funded trials involve collaboration between industry and academia, although academics are often not involved in the data analysis [100]. An evaluation of the research practices of the pharmaceutical industry led to the conclusion that 'those who have the gold make the evidence' [101].

In general drug company studies are at not at a higher risk of bias in methods than other trials [93], so the explanation for the higher frequency of positive results must lie elsewhere. Other possibilities have been suggested. These include the more frequent use of surrogate outcomes, and publication bias, in which trials with negative findings are not published [93, 102, 103]. An analysis of head-to-head trials (which directly compare drug versus drug, rather than drug versus placebo) showed that 96.5% of trials favoured the drug manufactured by the company funding the study [104]. This may provide evidence of industry manipulation. An analysis of internal documents from the industry found that suppression of negative studies and spinning of negative findings were recognised techniques [105]. As one author suggested, allowing drug companies to generate evidence 'is akin to letting a politician count their own votes' [103].

CONCLUSIONS

This chapter has explored the many sources of bias that commonly afflict randomised controlled trials. The randomised controlled trial is held to be the gold standard for evidence on treatment effectiveness, but that gold is more than a little tarnished. One commentator concluded that randomised controlled trials are: 'often flawed, mostly useless, clearly indispensable' [106].

The two key questions for clinical trials are: how frequently do these flaws occur; and how big an effect do they exert on estimated effect sizes? The frequency of flaws varies across individual review studies and by the type of deficiency, so there is not a specific estimate of how often bias occurs. Instead we can put the frequencies on a scale from very rare to very common. As most of the estimates from review articles are in the fairly common or very common area, flaws are a serious problem.

The magnitude of bias from randomisation and allocation concealment is generally modest, amounting to a 10%–15% increase in the estimated treatment effect. However these estimates are averages based on large numbers of trials that cover many different types of treatment. It is likely that the impact of bias is much larger for some trials than others, although we do not know which.

Some of the weaknesses in clinical trials may simply be due to lack of knowledge or experience. This could explain deficiencies in the handling loss to follow-up or the lack of blinding of outcome assessment. Tampering with the randomisation sequence, and the replacement of primary outcomes, suggests a less innocent explanation. The deficiencies described in this chapter, which may result from inadvertent mistakes or deliberate actions, pose a serious threat to the integrity of medical evidence. The next chapter describes weaknesses in study design and conduct that lead to wasted and unhelpful trials.

REFERENCES

1. Riechelmann, R.P., Peron, J., Seruga, B. et al. (2018). Meta-research on oncology trials: a toolkit for researchers with limited resources. *Oncologist* 23: 1467–1473.

2. Page, M.J., Higgins, J.P., Clayton, G. et al. (2016). Empirical evidence of study design biases in randomized trials: systematic review of meta-epidemiological studies. *PLoS One* https://doi.org/10.1371/journal.pone.0159267.

3. Adie, S., Harris, I.A., Naylor, J.M. et al. (2017). The quality of surgical versus non-surgical randomized controlled trials. *Contemp. Clin. Trials Commun.* 5: 63–66.

4. Savovic, J., Jones, H., Altman, D. et al. (2012). Influence of reported study design characteristics on intervention effect estimates from randomised controlled trials: combined analysis of meta-epidemiological studies. *Health Technol. Assess.* 16: 1–82.

5. Dechartres, A., Trinquart, L., Atal, I. et al. (2017). Evolution of poor reporting and inadequate methods over time in 20 920 randomised controlled trials included in Cochrane reviews: research on research study. *BMJ* https://doi.org/10.1136/bmj.j2490.

6. Wuytack, F., Regan, M., Biesty, L. et al. (2019). Risk of bias assessment of sequence generation: a study of 100 systematic reviews of trials. *Syst. Rev.* https://doi.org/10.1186/s13643-018-0924-1.

7. Savovic, J., Turner, R.M., Mawdsley, D. et al. (2018). Association between risk-of-bias assessments and results of randomized trials in Cochrane reviews: the ROBES meta-epidemiologic study. *Am. J. Epidemiol.* 187: 1113–1122.

8. Zhai, X., Cui, J., Wang, Y. et al. (2017). Quality of reporting randomized controlled trials in five leading neurology journals in 2008 and 2013 using the modified "risk of bias" tool. *World Neurosurg.* 99: 687–694.

9. Rikos, D., Dardiotis, E., Tsivgoulis, G. et al. (2016). Reporting quality of randomized-controlled trials in multiple sclerosis from 2000 to 2015, based on CONSORT statement. *Mult. Scler. Relat. Disord.* 9: 135–139.

10. Saltaji, H., Armijo-Olivo, S., Cummings, G.G. et al. (2018). Impact of selection bias on treatment effect size estimates in randomized trials of Oral health interventions: a meta-epidemiological study. *J. Dent. Res.* 97: 5–13.

11. Schulz, K.F. and Grimes, D.A. (2002). Unequal group sizes in randomised trials: guarding against guessing. *Lancet* 359: 966–970.

12. Clark, L., Fairhurst, C., Hewitt, C.E. et al. (2014). A methodological review of recent meta-analyses has found significant heterogeneity in age between randomized groups. *J. Clin. Epidemiol.* 67: 1016–1024.

13. Clark, L., Fairhurst, C., Cook, E. et al. (2015). Important outcome predictors showed greater baseline heterogeneity than age in two systematic reviews. *J. Clin. Epidemiol.* 68: 175–181.

14. Schulz, KF. (1995). Subverting randomization in controlled trials. *JAMA* 274: 1456–1458.

15. Paludan-Muller, A., Laursen, D.R.T., and Hrobjartsson, A. (2016). Mechanisms and direction of allocation bias in randomised clinical trials. *BMC Med. Res. Methodol.* https://doi.org/10.1186/s12874-016-0235-y.

16. Clark, L., Fairhurst, C., and Torgerson, D.J. (2016). Allocation concealment in randomised controlled trials: are we getting better? *BMJ* https://doi.org/10.1136/bmj.i5663.

17. Schulz, K.F., Chalmers, I., Hayes, R.J. et al. (1995). Empirical evidence of bias. Dimensions of methodological quality associated with estimates of treatment effects in controlled trials. *JAMA* 273: 408–412.

18. Dechartres, A., Trinquart, L., Faber, T. et al. (2016). Empirical evaluation of which trial characteristics are associated with treatment effect estimates. *J. Clin. Epidemiol.* 77: 24–37.

19. Pansieri, C., Pandolfini, C., and Bonati, M. (2015). The evolution in registration of clinical trials: a chronicle of the historical calls and current initiatives promoting transparency. *Eur. J. Clin. Pharmacol.* 71: 1159–1164.

20. Zarin, D.A., Tse, T., Williams, R.J. et al. (2017). Update on trial registration 11 years after the ICMJE policy was established. *N. Engl. J. Med.* 376: 383–391.

21. Howard, B., Scott, J.T., Blubaugh, M. et al. (2017). Systematic review: outcome reporting bias is a problem in high impact factor neurology journals. *PLoS One* https://doi.org/10.1371/journal.pone.0180986.

22. Wayant, C., Scheckel, C., Hicks, C. et al. (2017). Evidence of selective reporting bias in hematology journals: a systematic review. *PLoS One* https://doi.org/10.1371/journal.pone.0178379.

23. Hannink, G., Gooszen, H.G., and Rovers, M.M. (2013). Comparison of registered and published primary outcomes in randomized clinical trials of surgical interventions. *Ann. Surg.* 257: 818–823.

24. Raghav, K.P., Mahajan, S., Yao, J.C. et al. (2015). From protocols to publications: a study in selective reporting of outcomes in randomized trials in oncology. *J. Clin. Oncol.* 33: 3583–3590.

25. Dwan, K., Gamble, C., Williamson, P.R. et al. (2013). Systematic review of the empirical evidence of study publication bias and outcome reporting bias – an updated review. *PLoS One* https://doi.org/10.1371/journal.pone.0066844.

26. Li, G., Abbade, L.P.F., Nwosu, I. et al. (2018). A systematic review of comparisons between protocols or registrations and full reports in primary biomedical research. *BMC Med. Res. Methodol.* https://doi.org/10.1186/s12874-017-0465-7.

27. Chen, T., Li, C., Qin, R. et al. (2019). Comparison of clinical trial changes in primary outcome and reported intervention effect size between trial registration and publication. *JAMA Netw. Open* https://doi.org/10.1001/jamanetworkopen.2019.7242.

28. Smyth, R.M., Kirkham, J.J., Jacoby, A. et al. (2011). Frequency and reasons for outcome reporting bias in clinical trials: interviews with trialists. *BMJ* https://doi.org/10.1136/bmj.c7153.

29. van der Steen, J.T., van den Bogert, C.A., van Soest-Poortvliet, M.C. et al. (2018). Determinants of selective reporting: a taxonomy based on content analysis of a random selection of the literature. *PLoS One* https://doi.org/10.1371/journal.pone.0188247.

30. Bello, S., Moustgaard, H., and Hrobjartsson, A. (2017). Unreported formal assessment of unblinding occurred in 4 of 10 randomized clinical trials, unreported loss of blinding in 1 of 10 trials. *J. Clin. Epidemiol.* 81: 42–50.

31. Bello, S., Moustgaard, H., and Hrobjartsson, A. (2014). The risk of unblinding was infrequently and incompletely reported in 300 randomized clinical trial publications. *J. Clin. Epidemiol.* 67: 1059–1069.

32. Yi, J., Haibo, H.L., Li, Y. et al. (2020). Risk of bias and its impact on intervention effect estimates of randomized controlled trials in endodontics. *J. Endodontics* 46: 12–18.

33. Moustgaard, H., Clayton, G.L., Jones, H.E. et al. (2020). Impact of blinding on estimated treatment effects in randomised clinical trials: meta-epidemiological study. *BMJ* https://doi.org/10.1136/bmj.l6802.

34. Huupponen, R. and Viikari, J. (2013). Statins and the risk of developing diabetes. *BMJ* https://doi.org/10.1136/bmj.f3156.

35. Tang, E., Ravaud, P., Riveros, C. et al. (2015). Comparison of serious adverse events posted at http://ClinicalTrials.gov and published in corresponding journal articles. *BMC Med.* https://doi.org/10.1186/s12916-015-0430-4.

36. Favier, R. and Crepin, S. (2018). The reporting of harms in publications on randomized controlled trials funded by the "Programme Hospitalier de Recherche Clinique," a French academic funding scheme. *Clin. Trials* 15: 257–267.

37. Hughes, S., Cohen, D., and Jaggi, R. (2014). Differences in reporting serious adverse events in industry sponsored clinical trial registries and journal articles on antidepressant and antipsychotic drugs: a cross-sectional study. *BMJ Open* https://doi.org/10.1136/bmjopen-2014-005535.

38. Golder, S., Loke, Y.K., Wright, K. et al. (2016). Reporting of adverse events in published and unpublished studies of health care interventions: a systematic review. *PLoS Med.* https://doi.org/10.1371/journal.pmed.1002127.

39. Hodkinson, A., Kirkham, J.J., Tudur-Smith, C. et al. (2013). Reporting of harms data in RCTs: a systematic review of empirical assessments against the CONSORT harms extension. *BMJ Open* https://doi.org/10.1136/bmjopen-2013-003436.

40. Fewtrell, M.S., Kennedy, K., Singhal, A. et al. (2008). How much loss to follow-up is acceptable in long-term randomised trials and prospective studies? *Arch. Dis. Child.* 93: 458–461.

41. Schulz, K.F. and Grimes, D.A. (2002). Sample size slippages in randomised trials: exclusions and the lost and wayward. *Lancet* 359: 781–785.

42. Akl, E.A., Briel, M., You, J.J. et al. (2012). Potential impact on estimated treatment effects of information lost to follow-up in randomised controlled trials (LOST-IT): systematic review. *BMJ* https://doi.org/10.1136/bmj.e2809.

43. Zhang, Y., Florez, I.D., Colunga Lozano, L.E. et al. (2017). A systematic survey on reporting and methods for handling missing participant data for continuous outcomes in randomized controlled trials. *J. Clin. Epidemiol.* 88: 57–66.

44. Nuesch, E., Trelle, S., Reichenbach, S. et al. (2009). The effects of excluding patients from the analysis in randomised controlled trials: meta-epidemiological study. *BMJ* https://doi.org/10.1136/bmj.b3244.

45. Bell, M.L., Fiero, M., Horton, N.J. et al. (2014). Handling missing data in RCTs; a review of the top medical journals. *BMC Med. Res. Methodol.* https://doi.org/10.1186/1471-2288-14-118.

46. Walters, S.J., Bonacho Dos Anjos Henriques-Cadby, I., Bortolami, O. et al. (2017). Recruitment and retention of participants in randomised controlled trials: a review of trials funded and published by the United Kingdom Health Technology Assessment Programme. *BMJ Open* https://doi.org/10.1136/bmjopen-2016-015276.

47. Hussain, J.A., White, I.R., Langan, D. et al. (2016). Missing data in randomized controlled trials testing palliative interventions pose a

significant risk of bias and loss of power: a systematic review and meta-analyses. *J. Clin. Epidemiol.* 74: 57–65.

48. Ibrahim, F., Tom, B.D., Scott, D.L. et al. (2016). A systematic review of randomised controlled trials in rheumatoid arthritis: the reporting and handling of missing data in composite outcomes. *Trials* https://doi.org/10.1186/s13063-016-1402-5.

49. Miller, B.M. and Brennan, L. (2015). Measuring and reporting attrition from obesity treatment programs: a call to action! *Obes. Res. Clin. Pract.* 9: 187–202.

50. Marciniak, T.A., Cherepanov, V., Golukhova, E. et al. (2016). Drug discontinuation and follow-up rates in oral antithrombotic trials. *JAMA Intern. Med.* 176: 257–259.

51. Hussain, J.A., Bland, M., Langan, D. et al. (2017). Quality of missing data reporting and handling in palliative care trials demonstrates that further development of the CONSORT statement is required: a systematic review. *J. Clin. Epidemiol.* 88: 81–91.

52. White, I.R., Horton, N.J., Carpenter, J. et al. (2011). Strategy for intention to treat analysis in randomised trials with missing outcome data. *BMJ* https://doi.org/10.1136/bmj.d40.

53. Joseph, R., Sim, J., Ogollah, R. et al. (2015). A systematic review finds variable use of the intention-to-treat principle in musculoskeletal randomized controlled trials with missing data. *J. Clin. Epidemiol.* 68: 15–24.

54. Kahale, L.A., Diab, B., Khamis, A.M. et al. (2019). Potentially missing data are considerably more frequent than definitely missing data: a methodological survey of 638 randomized controlled trials. *J. Clin. Epidemiol.* 106: 18–31.

55. Altman, D.G. (2009). Missing outcomes in randomized trials: addressing the dilemma. *Open Med.* 3: 51–53.

56. Molnar, F.J., Hutton, B., and Fergusson, D. (2008). Does analysis using "last observation carried forward" introduce bias in dementia research? *CMAJ* 179: 751–753.

57. Lachin, J.M. (2016). Fallacies of last observation carried forward analyses. *Clin. Trials* 13: 161–168.

58. Lee, K.J. and Simpson, J.A. (2014). Introduction to multiple imputation for dealing with missing data. *Respirology* 19: 162–167.

59. Jakobsen, J.C., Gluud, C., Wetterslev, J. et al. (2017). When and how should multiple imputation be used for handling missing data in randomised clinical trials – a practical guide with flowcharts. *BMC Med. Res. Methodol.* https://doi.org/10.1186/s12874-017-0442-1.

60. Donders, A.R., van der Heijden, G.J., Stijnen, T. et al. (2006). Review: a gentle introduction to imputation of missing values. *J. Clin. Epidemiol.* 59: 1087–1091.

61. Montedori, A., Bonacini, M.I., Casazza, G. et al. (2011). Modified versus standard intention-to-treat reporting: are there differences in methodological quality, sponsorship, and findings in randomized trials? A cross-sectional study. *Trials* https://doi.org/10.1186/1745-6215-12-58.

62. Abraha, I., Cozzolino, F., Orso, M. et al. (2017). A systematic review found that deviations from intention-to-treat are common in randomized trials and systematic reviews. *J. Clin. Epidemiol.* 84: 37–46.

63. Abraha, I. and Montedori, A. (2010). Modified intention to treat reporting in randomised controlled trials: systematic review. *BMJ* https://doi.org/10.1136/bmj.c2697.

64. Abraha, I., Cherubini, A., Cozzolino, F. et al. (2015). Deviation from intention to treat analysis in randomised trials and treatment effect estimates: meta-epidemiological study. *BMJ* https://doi.org/10.1136/bmj.h2445.

65. Dossing, A., Tarp, S., Furst, D.E. et al. (2016). Modified intention-to-treat analysis did not bias trial results. *J. Clin. Epidemiol.* 72: 66–74.

66. Berger, V.W. (2017). Subjecting known facts to flawed empirical testing. *J. Clin. Epidemiol.* 84: 188.

67. Rainville, T., Laskine, M., and Durand, M. (2019). Use of modified intention-to-treat analysis in studies of direct oral anticoagulants and risk of selection bias: a systematic review. *BMJ Evid. Based Med.* 24: 63–69.

68. Farquhar, C.M., Showell, M.G., Showell, E.A.E. et al. (2017). Clinical trial registration was not an indicator for low risk of bias. *J. Clin. Epidemiol.* 84: 47–53.

69. Trinquart, L., Dunn, A.G., and Bourgeois, F.T. (2018). Registration of published randomized trials: a systematic review and meta-analysis. *BMC Med.* https://doi.org/10.1186/s12916-018-1168-6.

70. Odutayo, A., Emdin, C.A., Hsiao, A.J. et al. (2017). Association between trial registration and positive study findings: cross sectional study (epidemiological study of randomized trials-ESORT). *BMJ* https://doi.org/10.1136/bmj.j917.

71. Dechartres, A., Ravaud, P., Atal, I. et al. (2016). Association between trial registration and treatment effect estimates: a meta-epidemiological study. *BMC Med.* https://doi.org/10.1186/s12916-016-0639-x.

72. Nuesch, E., Trelle, S., Reichenbach, S. et al. (2010). Small study effects in meta-analyses of osteoarthritis trials: meta-epidemiological study. *BMJ* https://doi.org/10.1136/bmj.c3515.

73. Dechartres, A., Trinquart, L., Boutron, I. et al. (2013). Influence of trial sample size on treatment effect estimates: meta-epidemiological study. *BMJ* https://doi.org/10.1136/bmj.f2304.

74. Papageorgiou, S.N., Antonoglou, G.N., Tsiranidou, E. et al. (2014). Bias and small-study effects influence treatment effect estimates: a meta-epidemiological study in oral medicine. *J. Clin. Epidemiol.* 67: 984–992.

75. Pereira, T.V., Horwitz, R.I., and Ioannidis, J.P. (2012). Empirical evaluation of very large treatment effects of medical interventions. *JAMA* 308: 1676–1684.

76. Wang, Z., Alahdab, F., Almasri, J. et al. (2016). Early studies reported extreme findings with large variability: a meta-epidemiologic study in the field of endocrinology. *J. Clin. Epidemiol.* 72: 27–32.

77. Gartlehner, G., Dobrescu, A., Evans, T.S. et al. (2016). Average effect estimates remain similar as evidence evolves from single trials to high-quality bodies of evidence: a meta-epidemiologic study. *J. Clin. Epidemiol.* 69: 16–22.

78. Ioannidis, J.P. (2005). Contradicted and initially stronger effects in highly cited clinical research. *JAMA* 294: 218–228.

79. Ingre, M. (2013). Why small low-powered studies are worse than large high-powered studies and how to protect against "trivial" findings in research: comment on Friston (2012). *NeuroImage* 81: 496–498.

80. Walsh, M., Srinathan, S.K., McAuley, D.F. et al. (2014). The statistical significance of randomized controlled trial results is frequently fragile: a case for a fragility index. *J. Clin. Epidemiol.* 67: 622–628.

81. Ridgeon, E.E., Young, P.J., Bellomo, R. et al. (2016). The fragility index in multicenter randomized controlled critical care trials. *Crit. Care Med.* 44: 1278–1284.

82. Noel, C.W., McMullen, C., Yao, C. et al. (2018). The fragility of statistically significant findings from randomized trials in head and neck surgery. *Laryngoscope* 128: 2094–2100.

83. Evaniew, N., Files, C., Smith, C. et al. (2015). The fragility of statistically significant findings from randomized trials in spine surgery: a systematic survey. *Spine J.* 15: 2188–2197.

84. Mazzinari, G., Ball, L., Serpa Neto, A. et al. (2018). The fragility of statistically significant findings in randomised controlled anaesthesiology trials: systematic review of the medical literature. *Br. J. Anaesth.* 120: 935–941.

85. Edwards, E., Wayant, C., Besas, J. et al. (2018). How fragile are clinical trial outcomes that support the CHEST clinical practice guidelines for VTE? *Chest* 154: 512–520.

86. Lamberink, H.J., Otte, W.M., Sinke, M.R.T. et al. (2018). Statistical power of clinical trials increased while effect size remained stable: an empirical analysis of 136,212 clinical trials between 1975 and 2014. *J. Clin. Epidemiol.* 102: 123–128.

87. Colquhoun, D. (2014). An investigation of the false discovery rate and the misinterpretation of p-values. *R. Soc. Open Sci.* https://doi.org/10.1098/rsos.140216.

88. IntHout, J., Ioannidis, J.P., Borm, G.F. et al. (2015). Small studies are more heterogeneous than large ones: a meta-meta-analysis. *J. Clin. Epidemiol.* 68: 860–869.

89. Froud, R., Rajendran, D., Patel, S. et al. (2017). The power of low Back pain trials: a systematic review of power, sample size, and reporting of sample size calculations over time, in trials published between 1980 and 2012. *Spine* 42: E680–E686.

90. Azad, T.D., Veeravagu, A., Mittal, V. et al. (2018). Neurosurgical randomized controlled trials-distance travelled. *Neurosurgery* 82: 604–612.

91. Gan, H.K., You, B., Pond, G.R. et al. (2012). Assumptions of expected benefits in randomized phase III trials evaluating systemic treatments for cancer. *J. Natl. Cancer Inst.* 104: 590–598.

92. Matheson, A. (2017). Marketing trials, marketing tricks – how to spot them and how to stop them. *Trials* https://doi.org/10.1186/s13063-017-1827-5.

93. Lundh, A., Lexchin, J., Mintzes, B. et al. (2018). Industry sponsorship and research outcome: systematic review with meta-analysis. *Intensive Care Med.* 44: 1603–1612.

94. Riaz, H., Raza, S., Khan, M.S. et al. (2015). Impact of funding source on clinical trial results including cardiovascular outcome trials. *Am. J. Cardiol.* 116: 1944–1947.

95. Sismondo, S. (2008). Pharmaceutical company funding and its consequences: a qualitative systematic review. *Contemp. Clin. Trials* 29: 109–113.

96. Sturmberg, J.P. (2019). From probability to believability. *J. Eval. Clin. Pract.* 26: 1081–1086.

97. Smith, R. (2005). Medical journals are an extension of the marketing arm of pharmaceutical companies. *PLoS Med.* https://doi.org/10.1371/journal.pmed.0020138.

98. Pyke, S., Julious, S.A., Day, S. et al. (2011). The potential for bias in reporting of industry-sponsored clinical trials. *Pharm. Stat.* 10: 74–79.

99. Zwierzyna, M., Davies, M., Hingorani, A.D. et al. (2018). Clinical trial design and dissemination: comprehensive analysis of http://clinicaltrials.gov and PubMed data since 2005. *BMJ* https://doi.org/10.1136/bmj.k2130.

100. Rasmussen, K., Bero, L., Redberg, R. et al. (2018). Collaboration between academics and industry in clinical trials: cross sectional study of publications and survey of lead academic authors. *BMJ* https://doi.org/10.1136/bmj.k3654.

101. Lexchin, J. (2012). Those who have the gold make the evidence: how the pharmaceutical industry biases the outcomes of clinical trials of medications. *Sci. Eng. Ethics* 18: 247–261.

102. Dunn, A.G., Bourgeois, F.T., and Coiera, E. (2013). Industry influence in evidence production. *J. Epidemiol. Community Health* 67: 537–538.

103. Every-Palmer, S. and Howick, J. (2014). How evidence-based medicine is failing due to biased trials and selective publication. *J. Eval. Clin. Pract.* 20: 908–914.

104. Flacco, M.E., Manzoli, L., Boccia, S. et al. (2015). Head-to-head randomized trials are mostly industry sponsored and almost always favor the industry sponsor. *J. Clin. Epidemiol.* 68: 811–820.

105. Spielmans, G.I. and Parry, P.I. (2010). From evidence-based medicine to marketing-based medicine: evidence from internal industry documents. *J. Bioethic Inquiry* 7: 13–29.

106. Ioannidis, J.P.A. (2018). Randomized controlled trials: often flawed, mostly useless, clearly indispensable: a commentary on Deaton and cartwright. *Soc. Sci. Med.* 210: 53–56.

CHAPTER 3

Wasted and Unhelpful Trials

The volume of research evidence is truly immense, with tens of thousands of trials published annually [1]. Despite this, there are many fields of medicine in which evidence on treatment effectiveness is insufficient, sparse or absent [2–4]. The apparent contradiction between volume and scarcity can be explained by the poor quality of much research. A key paper by Chalmers and Glasziou in 2009 highlighted this problem, when they estimated that possibly as many as 85% of studies are wasted [5]. Much of the waste results from the types of bias that were explored in the previous chapter, but there are other causes. This chapter reviews the waste that results from other deficiencies in the research process. It also explores how some design features, particularly the choice and outcome measures and problems with generalisability, limit the value of trial results for clinical practice.

Evidence in Medicine: The Common Flaws, Why They Occur and How to Prevent Them,
First Edition. Iain K Crombie.
© 2021 John Wiley & Sons Ltd. Published 2021 by John Wiley & Sons Ltd.

WASTED STUDIES

Uncompleted Trials

On average, about one quarter of trials are stopped earlier than intended [6, 7]. The frequency of non-completion may vary between specialties, for example surgical trials were more likely to be uncompleted than medical ones (43% vs 27%) [8]. Failure to recruit patients is the most common cause of trials being abandoned: in three reviews, poor recruitment accounted for between 32% and 44% of discontinued trials [6, 7, 9]. A detailed investigation of this problem showed that, in most instances, careful planning and initial exploratory work could have prevented poor recruitment [10]. This failure to complete studies is a disservice to patients, and a waste of resources and the opportunity to evaluate treatment effectiveness.

Unpublished Trials

Many completed clinical trials are not published. This has been called the file drawer problem [11] in which completed studies are sometimes not reported in scientific journals. To identify the scale of the problem, researchers have identified several sources that register new trials such as: the funding bodies that supported them, the ethics committees that approved them, and international registries of trials. One review estimated that one third of trials are not published [12]. An overview of such reports found that the proportion of unpublished trials ranged from 14% to 76%, giving a pooled estimate of 46% [13]. There is strong evidence that unpublished studies are less likely to have significant findings and to have smaller effect sizes than published ones [13–15].

Several surveys have explored the reasons researchers do not publish their studies [16]. Many investigators mentioned lack of time or low priority (33%), unimportant or negative findings (12%) or fear of rejection by medical journals (12%). These explanations are consistent with the idea that researchers selectively publish 'wonderful results rather than negative results' [16], and often decide not to publish studies that have small effect sizes and non-significant results.

Unnecessary Trials

Some clinical trials are conducted when there is already clear evidence on the effectiveness of a treatment, and, as a result, many thousands of patients have been unnecessarily recruited to trials [17, 18]. Treatment of acute myocardial infarction with streoptokinase provides an early example of this type of waste [19]. The first 8 trials, involving 2,432 patients, confirmed that the drug significantly reduced mortality. This was followed by a further 25 trials and 34,542 patients, which made no difference to the estimated treatment benefit [19]. A more recent review examined this phenomenon for 13 treatments from across medicine [18]. The researchers found that there were wasted trials for eight of these treatments, such that between 12% and 89% of the patients involved had been unnecessarily recruited. Much waste could be avoided if researchers carefully reviewed previous research, to determine whether a new trial is needed [20]. In practice this may not be done. In published reports, about three quarters of previously published RCTs are not referenced [21], and many studies do not cite existing systematic reviews [22, 23].

NEGLECTED AREAS OF RESEARCH

Less Favoured Clinical Areas

Some clinical areas receive much less attention from research studies than their burden of ill health would merit. Research into mental health, stroke, injuries and chronic obstructive pulmonary disease (COPD) has suffered from serious underfunding [24–26]. Although cancer and coronary heart disease are usually well funded, there can be marked differences within these broad disease grouping. For example compared to the scale of disease, some types of cancer are well funded (e.g. breast, ovary and leukaemia) and others (e.g. lung, stomach and pancreas) receive much less funding [27].

Less Popular Types of Interventions

Evaluations of the effectiveness of drugs have dominated treatment research for decades. However, when asked, patients and clinicians strongly identify the need for non-drug therapies [28]. In cancer, patients want interventions that will help them deal with the practical, social and emotional issues resulting from their disease [29]. Patients with mental health problems identify stigma, discrimination and support for carers as the areas where interventions are needed [30]. The concentration of effort on drug research is not helping to meet the real needs of patients.

UNHELPFUL OUTCOME MEASURES

An important feature of effectiveness research is to decide how best to measure the benefits of the treatment i.e. which outcome measures to use. Ideally the outcome should be one that is likely to be influenced by the treatment, can be objectively, easily and reliably measured, and is relevant to patients and clinicians [31]. The chosen measure is often a compromise between these requirements. For many years ease of measurement and likelihood of detecting an effect were often prioritised over relevance to patients and clinicians. This led to the widespread use of two types of measure: surrogate and composite outcomes.

Surrogate Outcomes

Surrogate outcomes act as a substitute for clinically more important outcomes. They are widely used, particularly in surgery, diabetes care, glaucoma and cancer [32–35]. For example, in cancer treatment, shrinkage of the tumour and progression-free survival are commonly used as surrogates for overall patient survival [35]. The assumption is that the surrogates measure an intermediate step to a more important outcome (such as mortality). Surrogate measures are able to detect outcomes more quickly after treatment, and they can be measured on all patients (as opposed to death which only occurs in a few patients during a trial). This makes the measures very attractive: trials can be of shorter duration and fewer patients are needed, greatly reducing the costs.

In practice, surrogate measures are often poor predictors of the clinically important outcome. Many studies have demonstrated that there is only a weak relationship between surrogates and patient survival in cancer trials [36, 37]. Further, surrogate outcomes often lead to much larger estimates of benefit than is seen for more clinically relevant outcomes such as mortality [38]. In some instances, the surrogate outcomes can falsely suggest the treatment is beneficial. For example, the recent study of Venetoclax for multiple myeloma showed that the treatment was apparently beneficial when assessed by surrogate outcomes, but the death rate was twice as high in the treatment group than the control [39]. Surrogate measures need to be treated with great care.

Composite Outcomes

Composite outcomes combine two or more different measures into a single outcome. Many composite outcomes use three types of components: mortality, a clinical event (e.g. arrhythmia or respiratory distress) and a measure of healthcare usage (e.g. hospitalisation) [40]. These are combined into a single outcome measure, such that patients are counted as having experienced an event if they have suffered from one or more of the component measures.

Trials with composite outcomes are quicker and cheaper to conduct. This is because in many trials, the power of the study (ability to detect a significant effect) depends on the number of events that occur. Composite outcomes, which count the events occurring in any of the components, have large numbers of events and thus need smaller sample sizes. This benefit has encouraged the widespread use of composite outcomes in many medical fields including cardiovascular disease, rheumatology, nephrology and anaesthesia [40–42].

Despite their apparent advantages, composite outcomes have weaknesses. As Cordoba and colleagues [40] commented: 'composite outcomes are often unreasonably combined, inconsistently defined and inadequately reported'. For example, the definition of the composite may not be consistent across the abstract, the methods and the results section of the published paper [40]. The main problem with these measures is that the individual components of the composite may respond differently to the treatment, making the net effect of the composite difficult to interpret [43]. A good example of this is the impact of vitamin E on stroke. Although the treatment had no effect on the risk of total stroke, it significantly decreased the risk of ischaemic stroke and increased the risk of haemorrhagic stroke [44].

In general, if the benefit of the treatment is being driven by a less clinically important component of the composite (e.g. non-fatal arrhythmia as opposed to mortality), then the observed treatment effect size may be misleading. As one group commented, the composite outcome may provide 'an irrelevant average effect that does not represent any clinically meaningful effect' [43]. Composite outcomes should be treated with just as much care as surrogate measures.

Relevance to Patients and Clinicians

Trials with surrogate and composite outcomes have an additional limitation: their findings often 'fail to translate into benefits for patients' [45]. For example, patients may attach quite different importance to the elements of the composite outcome, valuing one much more than others [46]. Increasing emphasis is now being given to different types of outcome, those which are valued by patients and clinicians [46–48]. The concern is with 'how a patient feels, functions and survives' [31], rather than with biochemical or physiological measures. Outcomes that are important to patients are fatigue, depression, disability and ability to work [49, 50]. Patients also value interventions that give support for the practical, social and emotional issues arising from their illness [29]. These issues have often been given little attention [45, 47, 50], decreasing the value of the evidence many trials produce.

The use of composite outcomes has increased substantially in cardiovascular clinical trials, with a trend to increasing use of components of lesser clinical importance [51]. Many other clinical areas have seen a strong shift away from surrogate and composite outcome measures, with emphasis being put on patient relevant outcomes [45, 50, 52]. The core outcome measures in effectiveness trials (COMET) is helping to drive this much needed improvement in trial design.

COMET: Core Outcome Measures in Effectiveness Trials

Two important problems with trials are the diversity of outcomes used to evaluate individual treatments, and the lack of relevance of many outcomes for patients. In response, researchers began to develop sets of core outcomes for specific clinical conditions. This process is now coordinated by the COMET Initiative, which gives guidance on devising core outcomes and acts as a repository for existing outcome sets [53, 54]. Considerable progress has been made, with over 300 core outcome sets developed, although improvement is needed in some outcome sets [55]. A survey in 2017 found that patients had been involved in 87% of outcome measures under development [56]. The COMET handbook provides helpful guidance for those wishing to develop core outcome measures [57].

LACK OF GENERALISABILITY

An important factor limiting the value of trials in clinical practice is lack of generalisability (often termed external validity). This problem has been recognised for many years, but was highlighted by the phrase 'to whom do the results of this trial apply?' in a seminal paper by Rothwell [58]. Clinical trials often set restrictive entry criteria, so that many groups of patients are excluded from trials. Older patients [59–61] and those with more severe symptoms, poorer prognosis and multiple health problems [62–64] are often not recruited to trials. In the past women were also systematically excluded from trials [61] although this practice is gradually being abandoned [65].

The scale of exclusions of patients from trials is substantial, often exceeding 60% of the patients with the disease being treated [62, 66]. The result is that in most trials the patients treated are not representative of those seen in clinical practice [62]. As Cattadori and colleagues commented, trials in the US tend to recruit 'tall, white, blond-haired and blue-eyed, middle-aged, physically active, rich males' [67].

Possible Reasons for Exclusions

One reason for excluding some patients from a trial is to create a study group that will gain most benefit from the treatment and experience minimal side effects [68, 69]. Commonly, the groups that are excluded are less likely to benefit and to be more at risk of suffering adverse effects for several reasons. The elderly absorb and process medications differently from younger adults and this will affect the impact of medications [70]. Older patients are also at greater risk of adverse drug reactions [71, 72]. In addition patients with multiple health problems are more likely to suffer from poorer quality of life and are at an increased risk of dying [73]. Excluding high risk patients might ensure that they do not suffer harm from the treatment. But this could show a treatment in an inappropriately favourable light: in clinical practice all types of patients will be treated, so the overall benefit may be less than expected. The high frequency of exclusion of selected groups of patients (the elderly and those with comorbidities), could mean that the benefits of treatments seen in trials may not apply in routine clinical practice [64, 67, 74, 75].

Poor Reporting of Patient Characteristics

The challenge of generalisation is exacerbated by the poor reporting of patient characteristics. Among 196 trials in general practice only 40% reported the participants' comorbidities and 20% co-medications [75]. A similar problem is seen in trials focusing on older adults: physical and mental functioning, frailty and somatic status are under-reported to the extent that it is unclear 'to which older patients the results can be applied' [76]. Thus, for many if not most trials, it is unclear which types of patients are likely to benefit from the treatment.

The Average and the Individual

A clinical trial provides an estimate of the average treatment benefit occurring among trial participants. In reality some patients will gain considerable benefit while others may experience little benefit or even harm [77]. The problem is that doctors treat individuals, whereas trials deal with groups [78]. The limitations of applying average results to individual patients are widely recognised [79–81]. The development and testing of methods to identify which types of patients will benefit is a vibrant research area, covering stratified medicine, personalised medicine and precision medicine. These terms differ in the extent of matching to the individual, with stratified medicine using clinical characteristics [82] and precision medicine being based on genes, lifestyle and environment [83, 84]. The ultimate goal is to be able to identify the best treatment for the individual [82, 85, 86]. Enthusiasm for this approach is great, and there have been some initial successes, for example in the management of cystic fibrosis [83]; however, major advances in individualised therapy lie in the future [87].

WEAK AND MISLEADING EVIDENCE

Given the many problems with clinical trials described in this and the previous chapter, it is not surprising that some treatments are supported only by weak evidence. An analysis of new cancer drugs that were recently licensed for clinical use illustrates many of the problems with evidence [88]. Of the 54 studies that led to the drugs being approved for clinical use, 24% were not randomised controlled trials. Of the randomised studies, 74% used surrogate endpoints such as progression-free survival, even though such measures have only a low correlation with overall survival [37]. Further, 49% of these randomised trials were judged to be at high risk of bias, mainly due to concerns with the measurement of the outcome and missing outcome data [88]. Comparison of different source documents revealed inconsistencies in the reporting of study details. An editorial in a leading medical journal summed up the position with the title: 'flawed evidence underpins approval of new cancer drugs' [89].

Reversals in Medicine

Reversals in medicine occur when previously accepted treatments are withdrawn because subsequent large high quality studies show them to be ineffective or harmful [90]. A classic example is the use of corticosteroids for traumatic head injury. These drugs were thought to lower intracranial pressure and reduce death and disability. Although the evidence to support this view was limited, corticosteroids were widely used for head injury. A large well-conducted study then showed that the treatment was at best ineffective, and possibly harmful [91]; the drug may have caused over 2,500 unnecessary deaths before it was withdrawn [92].

Another example is a drug that was used to control arrhythmias in patients who had recently suffered a heart attack [93]. Cardiac arrhythmia is a very common cause of death in these patients, so controlling the heart rhythm was thought to be beneficial. In fact, this belief was so strongly held that the proposal to conduct a trial of the drug was widely considered to be unethical. Fortunately a trial was conducted to evaluate the effectiveness of the treatment. It showed that the drug caused an increased death rate. One estimate was that 50,000 American patients died during the time the drug was used [93].

These are not just isolated cases. One overview study examined trials published in one general medical journal over a 10 year period [90]. It found that 146 established treatments were subsequently shown to be ineffective. A more recent study, covering three leading medical journals, identified 396 medical reversals [94]. A common feature of these reversals is that the initial evidence to justify the use of the treatments was limited, being based on studies with weak methodology.

Lack of Reproducibility

Clinical trials of new drugs are undertaken when preclinical studies show that they have the potential to benefit patients. Serious concerns were raised about preclinical research when Begley and Ellis reported that, of 53 landmark preclinical studies in cancer research, the results of 47 could not be confirmed in subsequent studies. The finding that only 11% were reproducible was 'a shocking result' [95]. A recent symposium on preclinical research concluded that 'irreproducibility of biomedical research is a global issue' [96]. The problem is much wider than biomedicine: a survey of 1,576 researchers across science found that 52% believe that there is a reproducibility crisis [97]. Some commentators agree that science is facing a crisis [98, 99], although others take a different view [100]. Drug development will be hindered, and clinical trials will be wasted, because of the unreliability of preclinical research [95, 101].

CONCLUSION

Research waste was described as a scandal 25 years ago [102], and it is still a scandal today [103]. Possibly the only major change is that there is now greater awareness of the problem, and more insight into its nature [104, 105]. The causes of waste reside in all stages of the research process: from poor choice of research question, deficiencies in study design, flaws in study conduct, and in the writing up and publication of the findings [20, 105–107].

Research waste leads to uncertainties about the effects of treatments. Evidence is weak for patients with multiple health problems, particularly so for older people who are at high risk of having multiple morbidity. The problems of unpublished and poor quality research are compounded by the widespread use of surrogate and composite outcomes and the lack of generalisability of much completed research. The result is 'tens of thousands of uncertainties' about treatments [108]. The lack of convincing evidence for many current treatments is a serious issue for patients and those delivering healthcare.

The research community has responded to these challenges by launching a series of important initiatives to tackle research waste. These are listed in the Appendix 2, which also identifies many other proposals that have been made to improve the quality of medical research. Implementing these suggestions would involve major changes to the research environment, and would require substantial investment. The scale of the problem of research waste indicates that such drastic actions are essential.

REFERENCES

1. Viergever, R.F. and Li, K. (2015). Trends in global clinical trial registration: an analysis of numbers of registered clinical trials in different parts of the world from 2004 to 2013. *BMJ Open* https://doi.org/10.1136/bmjopen-2015-008932.

2. Villas Boas, P.J., Spagnuolo, R.S., Kamegasawa, A. et al. (2013). Systematic reviews showed insufficient evidence for clinical practice in 2004: what about in 2011? The next appeal for the evidence-based medicine age. *J. Eval. Clin. Pract.* 19: 633–637.

3. Sacco, P.C., Casaluce, F., Sgambato, A. et al. (2015). Current challenges of lung cancer care in an aging population. *Expert. Rev. Anticancer. Ther.* 15: 1419–1429.

4. Wilkinson, P., Ruane, C., and Tempest, K. (2018). Depression in older adults. *BMJ* https://doi.org/10.1136/bmj.k4922.

5. Chalmers, I. and Glasziou, P. (2009). Avoidable waste in the production and reporting of research evidence. *Lancet* 374: 86–89.

6. Kasenda, B., von Elm, E., You, J. et al. (2014). Prevalence, characteristics, and publication of discontinued randomized trials. *JAMA* 311: 1045–1051.

7. Chapman, S.J., Shelton, B., Mahmood, H. et al. (2014). Discontinuation and non-publication of surgical randomised controlled trials: observational study. *BMJ* https://doi.org/10.1136/bmj.g6870.

8. Rosenthal, R., Kasenda, B., Dell-Kuster, S. et al. (2015). Completion and publication rates of randomized controlled trials in surgery: an empirical study. *Ann. Surg.* 262: 68–73.

9. van den Bogert, C.A., Souverein, P.C., Brekelmans, C.T.M. et al. (2017). Recruitment failure and futility were the most common reasons for discontinuation of clinical drug trials. Results of a nationwide inception cohort study in the Netherlands. *J. Clin. Epidemiol.* 88: 140–147.

10. Briel, M., Olu, K.K., von Elm, E. et al. (2016). A systematic review of discontinued trials suggested that most reasons for recruitment failure were preventable. *J. Clin. Epidemiol.* 80: 8–15.

11. Rosenthal, R. (1979). The "file drawer" proble and tolerance for null results. *Psychol. Bull.* 86: 638–641.

12. Chen, R., Desai, N.R., Ross, J.S. et al. (2016). Publication and reporting of clinical trial results: cross sectional analysis across academic medical centers. *BMJ* https://doi.org/10.1136/bmj.i637.

13. Schmucker, C., Schell, L.K., Portalupi, S. et al. (2014). Extent of non-publication in cohorts of studies approved by research ethics committees or included in trial registries. *PLoS One* https://doi.org/10.1371/journal.pone.0114023.

14. Canestaro, W.J., Hendrix, N., Bansal, A. et al. (2017). Favorable and publicly funded studies are more likely to be published: a systematic review and meta-analysis. *J. Clin. Epidemiol.* 92: 58–68.

15. Dechartres, A., Atal, I., Riveros, C. et al. (2018). Association between publication characteristics and treatment effect estimates: a meta-epidemiologic study. *Ann. Intern. Med.* 169: 385–393.

16. Song, F., Loke, Y., and Hooper, L. (2014). Why are medical and health-related studies not being published? A systematic review of reasons given by investigators. *PLoS One* https://doi.org/10.1371/journal.pone.0110418.

17. Clarke, M., Brice, A., and Chalmers, I. (2014). Accumulating research: a systematic account of how cumulative meta-analyses would have provided knowledge, improved health, reduced harm and saved resources. *PLoS One* https://doi.org/10.1371/journal.pone.0102670.

18. Storz-Pfennig, P. (2017). Potentially unnecessary and wasteful clinical trial research detected in cumulative meta-epidemiological and trial sequential analysis. *J. Clin. Epidemiol.* 82: 61–70.

19. Lau, J., Antman, E.M., Jimenez-Silva, J. et al. (1992). Cumulative meta-analysis of therapeutic trials for myocardial infarction. *N. Engl. J. Med.* 327: 248–254.

20. Chalmers, I., Bracken, M.B., Djulbegovic, B. et al. (2014). How to increase value and reduce waste when research priorities are set. *Lancet* 383: 156–165.

21. Sawin, V.I. and Robinson, K.A. (2016). Biased and inadequate citation of prior research in reports of cardiovascular trials is a continuing source of waste in research. *J. Clin. Epidemiol.* 69: 174–178.

22. Rosenthal, R., Bucher, H.C., and Dwan, K. (2017). The use of systematic reviews when designing and reporting surgical trials. *Ann. Surg.* 265: e35–e36.

23. Engelking, A., Cavar, M., and Puljak, L. (2018). The use of systematic reviews to justify anaesthesiology trials: a meta-epidemiological study. *Eur. J. Pain* 22: 1844–1849.

24. Wykes, T., Haro, J.M., Belli, S.R. et al. (2015). Mental health research priorities for Europe. *Lancet Psychiatry* 2: 1036–1042.

25. Luengo-Fernandez, R., Leal, J., and Gray, A. (2015). UK research spend in 2008 and 2012: comparing stroke, cancer, coronary heart disease and dementia. *BMJ Open* https://doi.org/10.1136/bmjopen-2014-006648.

26. Gillum, L.A., Gouveia, C., Dorsey, E.R. et al. (2011). NIH disease funding levels and burden of disease. *PLoS One* https://doi.org/10.1371/journal.pone.0016837.

27. Carter, A.J., Delarosa, B., and Hur, H. (2015). An analysis of discrepancies between United Kingdom cancer research funding and societal burden and a comparison to previous and United States values. *Health Res. Policy Syst.* https://doi.org/10.1186/s12961-015-0050-7.

28. Crowe, S., Fenton, M., Hall, M. et al. (2015). Patients', clinicians' and the research communities' priorities for treatment research: there is an important mismatch. *Res. Involv. Engagem.* https://doi.org/10.1186/s40900-015-0003-x.

29. Corner, J., Wright, D., Hopkinson, J. et al. (2007). The research priorities of patients attending UK cancer treatment centres: findings from a modified nominal group study. *Br. J. Cancer* 96: 875–881.

30. Fiorillo, A., Luciano, M., Del Vecchio, V. et al. (2013). Priorities for mental health research in Europe: a survey among national stakeholders' associations within the ROAMER project. *World Psychiatry* 12: 165–170.

31. Fleming, T.R. and Powers, J.H. (2012). Biomarkers and surrogate endpoints in clinical trials. *Stat. Med.* 31: 2973–2984.

32. Adie, S., Harris, I.A., Naylor, J.M. et al. (2017). Are outcomes reported in surgical randomized trials patient-important? A systematic review and meta-analysis. *Can. J. Surg.* 60: 86–93.

33. Yudkin, J.S., Lipska, K.J., and Montori, V.M. (2011). The idolatry of the surrogate. *BMJ* https://doi.org/10.1136/bmj.d7995.

34. Yu, T., Hsu, Y.J., Fain, K.M. et al. (2015). Use of surrogate outcomes in US FDA drug approvals, 2003-2012: a survey. *BMJ Open* https://doi.org/10.1136/bmjopen-2015-007960.

35. Prasad, V. (2017). Do cancer drugs improve survival or quality of life? *BMJ* https://doi.org/10.1136/bmj.j4528.

36. Prasad, V., Kim, C., Burotto, M. et al. (2015). The strength of association between surrogate end points and survival in oncology: a systematic review of trial-level meta-analyses. *JAMA Intern. Med.* 175: 1389–1398.

37. Haslam, A., Hey, S.P., Gill, J. et al. (2019). A systematic review of trial-level meta-analyses measuring the strength of association between surrogate end-points and overall survival in oncology. *Eur. J. Cancer* 106: 196–211.

38. Ciani, O., Buyse, M., Garside, R. et al. (2015). Meta-analyses of randomized controlled trials show suboptimal validity of surrogate outcomes for overall survival in advanced colorectal cancer. *J. Clin. Epidemiol.* 68: 833–842.

39. Kumar, S. and Rajkumar, S.V. (2019). Surrogate endpoints in randomised controlled trials: a reality check. *Lancet* 394: 281–283.

40. Cordoba, G., Schwartz, L., Woloshin, S. et al. (2010). Definition, reporting, and interpretation of composite outcomes in clinical trials: systematic review. *BMJ* https://doi.org/10.1136/bmj.c3920.

41. Ibrahim, F., Tom, B.D., Scott, D.L. et al. (2016). A systematic review of randomised controlled trials in rheumatoid arthritis: the reporting and handling of missing data in composite outcomes. *Trials* https://doi.org/10.1186/s13063-016-1402-5.

42. Mascha, E.J. and Sessler, D.I. (2011). Statistical grand rounds: design and analysis of studies with binary- event composite endpoints: guidelines for anesthesia research. *Anesth. Analg.* 112: 1461–1471.

43. Prieto-Merino, D., Smeeth, L., Staa, T.P. et al. (2013). Dangers of non-specific composite outcome measures in clinical trials. *BMJ* https://doi.org/10.1136/bmj.f6782.

44. Schurks, M., Glynn, R.J., Rist, P.M. et al. (2010). Effects of vitamin E on stroke subtypes: meta-analysis of randomised controlled trials. *BMJ* https://doi.org/10.1136/bmj.c5702.

45. Heneghan, C., Goldacre, B., and Mahtani, K.R. (2017). Why clinical trial outcomes fail to translate into benefits for patients. *Trials* https://doi.org/10.1186/s13063-017-1870-2.

46. Stolker, J.M., Spertus, J.A., Cohen, D.J. et al. (2014). Rethinking composite end points in clinical trials: insights from patients and trialists. *Circulation* 130: 1254–1261.

47. Gaudry, S., Messika, J., Ricard, J.D. et al. (2017). Patient-important outcomes in randomized controlled trials in critically ill patients: a systematic review. *Ann. Intensive Care* https://doi.org/10.1186/s13613-017-0243-z.

48. Yordanov, Y., Dechartres, A., and Ravaud, P. (2018). Patient-important outcomes in systematic reviews: poor quality of evidence. *PLoS One* https://doi.org/10.1371/journal.pone.0195460.

49. Kirkham, J.J., Boers, M., Tugwell, P. et al. (2013). Outcome measures in rheumatoid arthritis randomised trials over the last 50 years. *Trials* https://doi.org/10.1186/1745-6215-14-324.

50. Williet, N., Sandborn, W.J., and Peyrin-Biroulet, L. (2014). Patient-reported outcomes as primary end points in clinical trials of inflammatory bowel disease. *Clin. Gastroenterol. Hepatol.* 12: 1246–56.e6.

51. Tan, N.S., Ali, S.H., Lebovic, G. et al. (2017). Temporal trends in use of composite end points in major cardiovascular randomized clinical trials in prominent medical journals. *Circ. Cardiovasc. Qual. Outcomes.*

52. Walton, M.K., Powers, J.H. 3rd, Hobart, J. et al. (2015). Clinical outcome assessments: conceptual foundation-report of the ISPOR clinical outcomes assessment – emerging good practices for outcomes research task force. *Value Health* 18: 741–752.

53. Gargon, E., Williamson, P.R., Altman, D.G. et al. (2017). The COMET initiative database: progress and activities update (2015). *Trials* https://doi.org/10.1186/s13063-017-1788-8.

54. Gargon, E., Williamson, P.R., and Young, B. (2017). Improving core outcome set development: qualitative interviews with developers provided pointers to inform guidance. *J. Clin. Epidemiol.* 86: 140–152.

55. Gargon, E., Williamson, P.R., Blazeby, J.M. et al. (2019). Improvement was needed in the standards of development for cancer core outcome sets. *J. Clin. Epidemiol.* 112: 36–44.

56. Biggane, A.M., Brading, L., Ravaud, P. et al. (2018). Survey indicated that core outcome set development is increasingly including patients, being conducted internationally and using Delphi surveys. *Trials* https://doi.org/10.1186/s13063-018-2493-y.

57. Williamson, P.R., Altman, D.G., Bagley, H. et al. (2017). The COMET handbook: version 1.0. *Trials* https://doi.org/10.1186/s13063-017-1978-4.

58. Rothwell, P.M. (2005). External validity of randomised controlled trials: "to whom do the results of this trial apply?". *Lancet* 365: 82–93.

59. Thake, M. and Lowry, A. (2017). A systematic review of trends in the selective exclusion of older participant from randomised clinical trials. *Arch. Gerontol. Geriatr.* 72: 99–102.

60. Bourgeois, F.T., Orenstein, L., Ballakur, S. et al. (2017). Exclusion of elderly people from randomized clinical trials of drugs for ischemic heart disease. *J. Am. Geriatr. Soc.* 65: 2354–2361.

61. Vitale, C., Fini, M., Spoletini, I. et al. (2017). Under-representation of elderly and women in clinical trials. *Int. J. Cardiol.* 232: 216–221.

62. Kennedy-Martin, T., Curtis, S., Faries, D. et al. (2015). A literature review on the representativeness of randomized controlled trial samples and implications for the external validity of trial results. *Trials* https://doi.org/10.1186/s13063-015-1023-4.

63. Boyd, C.M., Vollenweider, D., and Puhan, M.A. (2012). Informing evidence-based decision-making for patients with comorbidity: availability of necessary information in clinical trials for chronic diseases. *PLoS One* https://doi.org/10.1371/journal.pone.0041601.

64. Buffel du Vaure, C., Dechartres, A., Battin, C. et al. (2016). Exclusion of patients with concomitant chronic conditions in ongoing randomised controlled trials targeting 10 common chronic conditions and registered at http://ClinicalTrials.gov: a systematic review of registration details. *BMJ Open* https://doi.org/10.1136/bmjopen-2016-012265.

65. Pilote, L. and Raparelli, V. (2018). Participation of women in clinical trials: not yet time to rest on our laurels. *J. Am. Coll. Cardiol.* 71: 1970–1972.

66. Rothwell, P.M. (2006). Factors that can affect the external validity of randomised controlled trials. *PLoS Clin. Trials* https://doi.org/10.1371/journal.pctr.0010009.

67. Cattadori, G., Segurini, C., Agostoni, P. et al. (2018). A medicine for tall, white, blond-haired and blue-eyed, middle-aged, physically active, rich males? *Eur. J. Prev. Cardiol.* 25: 1152–1155.

68. Treweek, S. and Zwarenstein, M. (2009). Making trials matter: pragmatic and explanatory trials and the problem of applicability. *Trials* https://doi.org/10.1186/1745-6215-10-37.

69. Oude Rengerink, K., Kalkman, S., Collier, S. et al. (2017). Series: pragmatic trials and real world evidence: paper 3. Patient selection challenges and consequences. *J. Clin. Epidemiol.* 89: 173–180.

70. Brenes-Salazar, J.A., Alshawabkeh, L., Schmader, K.E. et al. (2015). Clinical pharmacology relevant to older adults with cardiovascular disease. *J. Geriatr. Cardiol.* 12: 192–195.

71. Davies, E.A. and O'Mahony, M.S. (2015). Adverse drug reactions in special populations – the elderly. *Br. J. Clin. Pharmacol.* 80: 796–807.

72. Anathhanam, S., Powis, R.A., Cracknell, A.L. et al. (2012). Impact of prescribed medications on patient safety in older people. *Ther. Adv. Drug. Saf.* 3: 165–174.

73. Gijsen, R., Hoeymans, N., Schellevis, F.G. et al. (2001). Causes and consequences of comorbidity: a review. *J. Clin. Epidemiol.* 54: 661–674.

74. Malmivaara, A. (2019). Generalizability of findings from randomized controlled trials is limited in the leading general medical journals. *J. Clin. Epidemiol.* 107: 36–41.

75. Braend, A.M., Straand, J., and Klovning, A. (2017). Clinical drug trials in general practice: how well are external validity issues reported? *BMC Fam. Pract.* 18: 113. https://doi.org/10.1186/s12875-017-0680-7.

76. van Deudekom, F.J., Postmus, I., van der Ham, D.J. et al. (2017). External validity of randomized controlled trials in older adults, a systematic review. *PLoS One* https://doi.org/10.1371/journal.pone.0174053.

77. Varadhan, R., Segal, J.B., Boyd, C.M. et al. (2013). A framework for the analysis of heterogeneity of treatment effect in patient-centered outcomes research. *J. Clin. Epidemiol.* 66: 818–825.

78. Dahabreh, I.J., Hayward, R., and Kent, D.M. (2016). Using group data to treat individuals: understanding heterogeneous treatment effects in the age of precision medicine and patient-centred evidence. *Int. J. Epidemiol.* 45: 2184–2193.

79. Kravitz, R.L., Duan, N., and Braslow, J. (2004). Evidence-based medicine, heterogeneity of treatment effects, and the trouble with averages. *Milbank Q.* 82: 661–687.

80. Kent, D.M. and Hayward, R.A. (2007). Limitations of applying summary results of clinical trials to individual patients: the need for risk stratification. *JAMA* 298: 1209–1212.

81. Davidoff, F. (2017). Can knowledge about heterogeneity in treatment effects help us choose wisely? *Ann. Intern. Med.* 166: 141–142.

82. Fisher, D.J., Carpenter, J.R., Morris, T.P. et al. (2017). Meta-analytical methods to identify who benefits most from treatments: daft, deluded, or deft approach? *BMJ* https://doi.org/10.1136/bmj.j573.

83. Ashley, E.A. (2015). The precision medicine initiative: a new national effort. *JAMA* 313: 2119–2120.

84. Hodson, R. (2016). Precision medicine. *Nature* 537: S49.

85. Herman, W.H., Pan, Q., Edelstein, S.L. et al. (2017). Impact of lifestyle and metformin interventions on the risk of progression to diabetes and regression to normal glucose regulation in overweight or obese people with impaired glucose regulation. *Diabetes Care* 40: 1668–1677.

86. Kent, D.M., Steyerberg, E., and van Klaveren, D. (2018). Personalized evidence based medicine: predictive approaches to heterogeneous treatment effects. *BMJ* https://doi.org/10.1136/bmj.k4245.

87. Khoury, M.J. and Galea, S. (2016). Will precision medicine improve population health? *JAMA* 316: 1357–1358.

88. Naci, H., Davis, C., Savovic, J. et al. (2019). Design characteristics, risk of bias, and reporting of randomised controlled trials supporting approvals of cancer drugs by European medicines agency, 2014-16: cross sectional analysis. *BMJ* https://doi.org/10.1136/bmj.l5221.

89. Mintzes, B. and Vitry, A. (2019). Flawed evidence underpins approval of new cancer drugs. *BMJ* https://doi.org/10.1136/bmj.l5399.

90. Prasad, V., Vandross, A., Toomey, C. et al. (2013). A decade of reversal: an analysis of 146 contradicted medical practices. *Mayo Clin. Proc.* 88: 790–798.

91. Edwards, P., Arango, M., Balica, L. et al. (2005). Final results of MRC CRASH, a randomised placebo-controlled trial of intravenous corticosteroid in adults with head injury-outcomes at 6 months. *Lancet* 365: 1957–1959.

92. Sauerland, S. and Maegele, M. (2004). A CRASH landing in severe head injury. *Lancet* 364: 1291–1292.

93. Prasad, V. and Cifu, A. (2013). The reversal of cardiology practices: interventions that were tried in vain. *Cardiovasc. Diagn. Ther.* 3: 228–235.

94. Herrera-Perez, D., Haslam, A., Crain, T. et al. (2019). A comprehensive review of randomized clinical trials in three medical journals reveals 396 medical reversals. *elife* https://doi.org/10.7554/eLife.45183.

95. Begley, C.G. and Ellis, L.M. (2012). Drug development: raise standards for preclinical cancer research. *Nature* 483: 531–533.

96. Anonymous (2015). *Reproducibility and reliability of biomedical research: improving research practice.* Symposium report. Academy of Medical Sciences, BBSRC, MRC, Wellcome Trust. https://acmedsci.ac.uk/file-download/38189-56531416e2949.pdf (accessed 10 October 2020).

97. Baker, M. (2016). 1,500 scientists lift the lid on reproducibility. *Nature* 533: 452–454.

98. Franca, T.F.A. and Monserrat, J.M. (2019). Reproducibility crisis, the scientific method, and the quality of published studies: untangling the knot. *Learned Publishing* 32: 406–408.

99. Munafo, M.R., Nosek, B.A., Bishop, D.V.M. et al. A manifesto for reproducible science. *Nat. Hum. Behav.* 2017 https://doi.org/10.1038/s41562-016-0021.

100. Fanelli, D. (2018). Is science really facing a reproducibility crisis, and do we need it to? *Proc. Natl Acad. Sci. USA* 115: 2628–2631.

101. Eisner, D.A. (2018). Reproducibility of science: fraud, impact factors and carelessness. *J. Mol. Cell. Cardiol.* 114: 364–368.

102. Altman, D.G. (1994). The scandal of poor medical research. *BMJ* https://doi.org/10.1136/bmj.308.6924.283.

103. Glasziou, P. and Chalmers, I. (2018). Research waste is still a scandal-an essay by Paul Glasziou and Iain Chalmers. *BMJ* https://doi.org/10.1136/bmj.k4645.

104. Ioannidis, J.P. (2014). Clinical trials: what a waste. *BMJ* https://doi.org/10.1136/bmj.g7089.

105. Moher, D., Glasziou, P., Chalmers, I. et al. (2016). Increasing value and reducing waste in biomedical research: who's listening? *Lancet* 387: 1573–1586.

106. Ioannidis, J.P., Greenland, S., Hlatky, M.A. et al. (2014). Increasing value and reducing waste in research design, conduct, and analysis. *Lancet* 383: 166–175.

107. Glasziou, P., Altman, D.G., Bossuyt, P. et al. (2014). Reducing waste from incomplete or unusable reports of biomedical research. *Lancet* 383: 267–276.

108. Chalmers, I., Atkinson, P., Fenton, M. et al. (2013). Tackling treatment uncertainties together: the evolution of the James Lind initiative, 2003–2013. *J. R. Soc. Med.* 106: 482–491.

CHAPTER 4

Can the Analysis Bias the Findings?

The analysis of the clinical data is an exciting stage of a trial, answering the key question: could the new treatment be effective? For many researchers, the focus is on statistical significance, and whether the p-value is less or greater than 0.05. Below this threshold the trial is celebrated as a success, but above it the treatment is deemed a failure. The p-value has become the statistical equivalent of a 'Seal of Good Housekeeping' [1].

The exclusive focus on statistical significance makes statisticians shudder, because p-values make a limited contribution to the evaluation of effectiveness. The assessment should take into account other factors including the size of treatment effect, the precision of the estimate, the consistency of the results, potential sources of bias in the study and the biological plausibility of the finding [2, 3]. Concentrating on the p-value is an example of using statistics 'as a drunken man uses lamp-posts – for support rather than illumination' (attributed to Lang, cited in Sturmberg [4]).

Evidence in Medicine: The Common Flaws, Why They Occur and How to Prevent Them, First Edition. Iain K Crombie.
© 2021 John Wiley & Sons Ltd. Published 2021 by John Wiley & Sons Ltd.

This chapter explores the role of p-values and the way they are misused. It will also describe the ways in which the analysis can be manipulated to create the chrysalis effect: turning ugly data into a beautiful finding [5]. Other more explicit terms for this process, such as p-hacking [6] and data ransacking [7], convey the appropriate sense of the brutal mishandling of the data and its analysis. As Mills remarked 'If you torture the data long enough they will tell you what you want to hear' [8]. The unrestrained quest for a significant p-value underlies many of the problems with medical research.

THE P-VALUE PROBLEM

P-values are extremely common in medical research, with the convention that $p \leq 0.05$ designates statistical significance. One study explored the p-values in the text of thousands of papers listed in Medline and PubMed Central from 1990 to 2015. Of the articles that presented a p-value, 96% had at least one result with $p \leq 0.05$ [9]. A complementary study found that 94% of the p-values in tables and figures were statistically significant [10]. Together these studies suggest there is a remarkably high frequency of significant results.

The major problem with the p-value is the 'widespread, mistaken belief' that it provides a rule 'for separating the true and important from the untrue or unimportant' [11]. P-values were never intended to provide a decision rule, but simply to provide an informal method to identify findings that were 'worthy of a second look' [12]. Now, as an editorial in the leading American statistics journal commented, 'the tool has become the tyrant' [13]. For clinical trials this simplistic decision rule leads to treatments being labelled as being effective or ineffective, a false dichotomisation of evidence [14]. In response to widespread concern, the American Statistical Association's guidance on p-values concluded with the statement: 'no single index should substitute for scientific reasoning' [15]. Clearly there is little difference between the $p = 0.049$ and $p = 0.051$, making it somewhat bizarre that one value would lead to a treatment being used in medicine while the other to it being discarded.

Definition of the P-value

The difficulty of describing statistical tests and p-values is that there are 'no interpretations of these concepts that are at once simple, intuitive, correct and foolproof' [16]. The following definition is intended to be straightforward, involving an explanation followed by some qualifications. The p-value is: the probability that the observed effect size, or a more extreme one, could occur if the null hypothesis is true [17]. The null hypothesis in clinical trials is usually that the treatments are equally effective (i.e. that one is not better than the other). The definition also assumes that the assumptions made by the statistical model are met (e.g. that the data points are independent and follow a defined distribution such as the normal distribution).

The important point is that the p-value gives the probability that the result is due to chance (if the null hypothesis of no effect is true and the requirements of the statistical model are met). In general, a p-value of $p \leq 0.05$ will occur by chance about once for every 20 (independent) statistical tests conducted. Carry out enough statistical tests on a data set, and you will eventually stumble on a spuriously significant result.

The Frequency of Reported P-values

The misplaced emphasis on statistical significance has an interesting effect on the frequency of reported p-values. A review of 2,000 Medline abstracts found that there were many more p-values just below 0.05 as there were just above 0.05 [18]. Thus, findings that are just significant appear to occur much more commonly than those which are just non-significant. This result has been replicated by other studies [19, 20], with one study reporting that the preponderance of p-values below 0.05 has increased over time [21]. A similar pronounced excess of p-values just below the threshold has been found at the other levels of statistical significance: highly significant ($p < 0.01$), and very highly significant ($p < 0.001$) [22]. As Gadbury has suggested, there may be 'inappropriate fiddling with statistical analyses to obtain a desirable p-value' [23].

Another possible explanation for the excess of p-values just below the thresholds is publication bias: studies with significant findings are more likely to be published than those whose findings are non-significant. There is substantial evidence for publication bias [24–26], and this could explain at least part of the excess of p-values just below 0.05. However, it cannot easily explain the similar effects seen at $p < 0.01$ and $p < 0.001$, as studies with p-values below 0.05 are likely to be published. The more plausible explanation is the deliberate, even if well-intentioned, push of 'a near significant p-value to a level that is considered significant' [23]. There is evidence that this happens: surveys have shown that between 3% and 23% of researchers admit to rounding down p-values [27–29].

Calculating and Reporting P-values

Problems frequently occur in the use of statistical tests. One review of the reporting of statistical methods found that 'a high percentage of articles contain errors in the application, analysis, interpretation, or reporting of statistics or in the design or conduct of research' [30]. For example, the frequencies of the use of inappropriate statistical methods ranged from 37% for orthopaedic studies [31] to 47% of papers submitted to the journal *Injury* [32]. A separate review reported that in 50% of papers examined, the stated p-values were inconsistent with the reported statistical test details (test statistic and degrees of freedom) [33]. These inconsistencies occurred more often when the reported p-value was <0.05, suggesting that some cases of misreporting may not have been accidental.

QUESTIONABLE RESEARCH PRACTICES

Questionable research practices refer to a variety of techniques that could 'spuriously increase the likelihood of finding evidence in support of a hypothesis' [29]. There are many of them, and their use is widespread throughout science [6]. Sacco and colleagues have produced a list of 31 these techniques [34]; those most likely to result in biased estimates of treatment benefit are described below.

HARKing (Hypothesising After the Results are Known)

Exploratory analyses of data is a process of repeatedly looking at data to see if they contain something interesting. This can be a valuable practice, but it can go wrong when a serendipitous finding is presented as if it were the main study hypothesis. Presenting a significant post hoc finding as an a priori hypothesis is known as HARKing [35]. It relies on a feature of p-values: if enough statistical tests are carried out, a spuriously significant result will eventually be found. Many non-significant results will be generated during the search, but these can be quietly buried. HARKing may be a common practice: a survey of biomedical scientists found that 20% had reported an unexpected finding as if it had been a prior hypothesis [36].

Excluding Data

Another questionable technique is to exclude a few measurements (data points) without giving an explanation of why this has been done. This technique has a long history. Charles Babbage, in his 1830 book on the decline of science, is critical of a method of cooking to make the data fit the theory. In this the researcher would 'make multitudes of observations, and out of these to select those only which agree, or very nearly agree' (cited by Jennings [37]). An initial analysis would identify the unhelpful data points, which would be excluded from a second analysis. This may be a common practice today. In one study, 15% of researchers admitted that they had excluded selected data points based on gut feeling [38], and in another study 13% did so after looking at the results [27].

Multiple Comparisons

Research studies often conduct and report several tests of significance. For example, among papers published in orthopaedic journals, 30% conducted more than 20 statistical tests and one reported 156 tests [31]. The problem is that multiple testing increases the risk of spurious significance. (Technically it inflates the type I error rate, the probability of rejecting the null hypothesis.) A good illustration of this was a fictional study investigating the link between the consumption of jelly babies and acne [39]. Overall there was no increase in the risk of acne, but, when 20 different colours were tested separately, one, the green one, had a statistically significant association with acne ($p < 0.05$). In the absence of any other evidence that green jelly babies exert some malign influence, this finding can be dismissed as nonsense.

Another example, using real data, explored the association between astrological sign and common diagnoses among hospitalised patients [40]. No prior hypotheses were stated. Instead each of the 12 star signs was tested against 223 different causes of hospitalisation. The authors were able to identify spuriously significant findings for each star sign: for example Saggitarians were at a higher risk of fractures of the humerus whereas those born under Leo were more likely to have gastrointestinal haemorrhage [40].

Multiple testing can occur in trials that have several outcome measures [41]. Among trials in neurology and psychiatry, 29% had more than one primary outcome measure [42], whereas 47% of trials in depression had at least two and 25% had at least five primary outcomes [43]. Many of these studies also included several secondary outcomes, giving considerable opportunity for multiple testing. The actual number of outcomes analysed may be higher than those stated in published reports, as the outcome measures listed in protocols are frequently replaced by new ones in the final report [44, 45]. Statistical methods to adjust for the increased risk of spurious significance are available [41, 46], but these are seldom used [42, 43, 47]. Multiple testing in trials remains a serious problem.

Subgroup Analyses

Subgroup analyses explore whether certain types of patients are more likely to gain benefit from a treatment (e.g. whether younger patients or those with less severe illness gain more benefit from treatment). This could enable therapies to be targeted to individuals, so it is not surprising that almost 50% of published clinical trials conduct subgroup analyses [48]. One investigation of this found that when trials conduct these analyses, 30% made claims about the effectiveness of the treatment in at least one subgroup [49]. Another review found that among 64 trials, a total of 117 subgroup claims were made [50]. These analyses need to be treated with caution because they are very likely to produce misleading results [51]. The sample size of a subgroup is much smaller than for the whole trial, and this reduces the power to detect treatment benefits. Further, because these analyses involve multiple comparisons, they are more likely to encounter spurious significance [52].

To protect against these potential problems, formal guidance describes when and how to conduct and interpret subgroup analyses [53]. Before subgroup analyses are conducted, a test of interaction should be conducted. This explores whether, overall, there is evidence (statistical significance) that one or more of the groups has a different effects size to the combined estimated. (The term interaction means that the treatment acts differently in some subgroups than in others.) One assessment found that among trials that carried out subgroup analyses, only 28% reported the test for interaction [50].

Another requirement for subgroup analysis is prespecification of the proposed analysis [53] (e.g. in the study protocol): this was reported in fewer than one half of trials [48, 54]. Further, in over one third of studies that reported they had prespecified the analysis, these details were absent from the protocols [48]. Subgroup analyses are often deeply flawed, and it seems advisable to follow Peter Sleight's guidance that they are 'fun to look at, but don't believe them' [55]. Only when a specific subgroup has been nominated in advance, a convincing scientific rationale is given for it, and the appropriate test for interaction has been conducted, can such analyses be taken seriously.

Selection of Covariates

Covariates are factors such as patient age or disease severity, which could affect the primary outcome of a trial. Although on average randomisation will produce two groups that are balanced at baseline, in practice small differences will often occur between the groups.

Adjusting for these baseline factors (covariates) ensures that the estimated treatment effect is not influenced by any small imbalances at baseline [56, 57]. The adjustment can also increase the power of the study. It is recommended that only a small number of covariates, those that are strongly predictive of the outcome, should be included in the analysis [58]. The covariates to be used should be prespecified, to prevent bias being introduced by choices made during the analysis [58]. The CONSORT statement for reporting of trials recommends that both unadjusted and adjusted analyses be presented [59].

One danger is that covariates are selected for inclusion in the analysis because they make the results look better (i.e. significant). Researchers could run several analyses with different combinations of covariates, choosing the set that gave the desired result. A simulation study showed that careful selection of covariates could increase the observed effect size: the average increase was 8%, but this rose to 58% in small trials [60]. A motivated selection of covariates may occur in practice: in a review of 200 trials, Saquib and colleagues found that the chosen covariates differed from those prespecified in the protocol in 47% of trials [61]. Choices about the covariate analyses can influence the size and statistical significance of treatment effects.

ENSURING HIGH QUALITY ANALYSIS: THE STATISTICAL ANALYSIS PLAN

To prevent questionable research practices, a Statistical Analysis Plan should be prepared before the analysis is begun: ideally it should be published in a journal or included in the entry to an international trial registry. It provides a detailed, technical description of the analyses that will be carried out and should be written and dated, and signed by the trial leader and the statistician [62]. The document should cover: the statistical methods, the primary and secondary outcomes, and the covariates for which adjustment will be made. It should also specify any subgroup analyses, as well as the approach for dealing with missing data. Some of the information on the proposed analysis may be presented in study protocols, but these documents may not provide sufficient detail: a review of 99 protocols found that only 27% specified the statistical method, 40% defined the covariates and 10% had a strategy for handling missing data [63].

The idea behind the plan is to prevent any temptation to manipulate the data analysis, by declaring in advance what will be done. Making the document publicly available should give reassurance that the analyses described in any report or publication are those that were planned. This may not always be the case. Overviews of review studies show that discrepancies frequently occur between the prespecified analyses and those presented in published papers [45, 64]. For example, changes in the use of covariates occurred in 46% up to 82% of trials; and 12%–100% for handling of subgroup analyses [45, 64]. Some, or indeed all, of these changes may have been made for legitimate reasons, but explanations for the discrepancies were not given in the trial reports. When not accounted for, these changes raise concern that the analyses have been deliberately manipulated. Methods of ensuring adherence to the pre-specified analysis may be required.

CONCLUSIONS

This chapter has described the problems caused by an overly simplistic decision rule that leads to an undignified chase for statistical significance. Almost all published articles present significant findings [9, 10], to the extent that negative results are disappearing from journals [65]. A curious feature of this phenomenon is that while the frequency of significant findings is rising, the reported effect sizes are diminishing [66]. In general, smaller effect sizes are 'likely to lead to a loss of statistical significance' [66]. This led the authors of this work to wonder whether an increasing emphasis on novelty and sensationalism might explain the divergence in trends between statistical significance and effect size.

The preponderance of p-values just below conventional thresholds indicates that something is amiss. It is clear that statistical analysis often fails to follow accepted practice, and is sometimes deliberately manipulated. Many researchers believe, possibly correctly, that a p-value of less than 0.05 increases the chances of publication in a high quality journal. This provides the incentive to tamper with the study design, or manipulate the data analysis, to obtain statistical significance. Many dubious statistical practices provide the means to meddle with p-values. This view is supported by a survey of consulting statisticians, which found that many had received requests that constituted extreme violations of good statistical practice [67]. For example 24% had been asked to remove or alter data records, 30% to interpret the findings to fit expectations rather than results, 29% to ignore violations of test assumptions because they led to non-significant findings, and 16% to stress significant findings while under-reporting non-significant ones. A follow-up paper described other unacceptable requests: only report results from a subset of the data (51%), analyse data when the randomisation sequence had been altered (22%), give a biased interpretation of a statistical finding (44%) and analyse data that were at least partly fabricated (14%) [68].

Researchers often have free rein to conduct extensive analyses in the search for a hypothesis with a significant finding. These include the choice of statistical tests, the treatment of outliers, the selection of covariates and the use of subgroup analysis. Collectively these are known as researcher degrees of freedom [69]. Forstmeier and colleagues liken these degrees of freedom to a walk through a garden of forking paths, with 'a near-endless diversity of combinations of decision variants' [70]: each choice may have a small effect, but cumulatively they could lead to quite different findings. Evidence for this comes from reanalyses of data from clinical trials: of 37 studies, the reanalysis led to differing conclusions in 13 (35%) of the trials [71]. Many of the techniques for statistical sleight of hand could be detected, and possibly prevented, through a Statistical Analysis Plan. Prepublication of this should encourage honest analysis, and aid the detection of delinquent behaviour.

In summary the statistical analysis, and statistical significance, should be part of a fair and balanced assessment of treatment effectiveness. In practice, flaws in the analyses are common, and some of them may result from a deliberate attempt to distort the true value of treatments. There is much truth in a pithy remark widely attributed to Aaron Levenstein: 'Statistics are like a bikini. What they reveal is suggestive, but what they conceal is vital'. Or, as Colquhoun wrote more recently, 'the function of significance tests is to prevent you from making a fool of yourself, and not to make unpublishable results publishable' [72].

REFERENCES

1. Cutler, S.J., Greenhouse, S.W., Cornfield, J. et al. (1966). The role of hypothesis testing in clinical trials. Biometrics seminar. *J Chronic Dis.* 19: 857–882.

2. Gagnier, J.J. and Morgenstern, H. (2017). Misconceptions, misuses, and misinterpretations of P values and significance testing. *J. Bone Joint Surg. Am.* 99: 1598–1603.

3. Lytsy, P. (2018). P in the right place: revisiting the evidential value of P-values. *J. Evid. Based Med.* 11: 288–291.

4. Sturmberg, J. and Topolski, S. (2014). For every complex problem, there is an answer that is clear, simple and wrong: and other aphorisms about medical statistical fallacies. *J. Eval. Clin. Pract.* 20: 1017–1025.

5. O'Boyle, E.H., Banks, G.C., and Gonzalez-Mule, E. (2017). The Chrysalis effect: how ugly initial results Metamorphosize into beautiful articles. *Aust. J. Manag.* 43: 376–399.

6. Head, M.L., Holman, L., Lanfear, R. et al. (2015). The extent and consequences of p-hacking in science. *PLoS Biol.* https://doi.org/10.1371/journal.pbio.1002106.

7. Suter, W.N. and Suter, P.M. (2015). How research conclusions go wrong: a primer for home health clinicians. *Home Health Care Manag. Pract.* 27: 171–177.

8. Mills, J.L. (1993). Data torturing. *N. Engl. J. Med.* 329: 1196–1199.

9. Chavalarias, D., Wallach, J.D., Li, A.H. et al. (2016). Evolution of reporting P values in the biomedical literature, 1990–2015. *JAMA* 315: 1141–1148.

10. Cristea, I.A. and Ioannidis, J.P.A. (2018). P values in display items are ubiquitous and almost invariably significant: a survey of top science journals. *PLoS One* https://doi.org/10.1371/journal.pone.0197440.

11. Mark, D.B., Lee, K.L., and Harrell, F.E. Jr. (2016). Understanding the role of P values and hypothesis tests in clinical research. *JAMA Cardiol.* 1: 1048–1054.

12. Nuzzo, R. (2014). Statistical errors. *Nature* 506: 150–152.

13. Wasserstein, R.L., Schirm, A.L., and Lazar, N.A. (2019). Moving to a world beyond "p < 0.05". *Am. Stat.* 73: 1–19.

14. McShane, B.B. and Gal, D. (2017). Statistical significance and the dichotomization of evidence. *J. Am. Stat. Assoc.* 112: 885–895.

15. Wasserstein, R.L. and Lazar, N.A. (2016). The ASA's statement on p-values: context, process, and purpose. *Am. Stat.* 70: 129–131.

16. Greenland, S., Senn, S.J., Rothman, K.J. et al. (2016). Statistical tests, P values, confidence intervals, and power: a guide to misinterpretations. *Eur. J. Epidemiol.* 31: 337–350.

17. Goodman, S.N. (1999). Toward evidence-based medical statistics. 1: the P value fallacy. *Ann. Intern. Med.* 130: 995–1004.

18. Ginsel, B., Aggarwal, A., Xuan, W. et al. (2015). The distribution of probability values in medical abstracts: an observational study. *BMC Res. Notes* https://doi.org/10.1186/s13104-015-1691-x.

19. Masicampo, E.J. and Lalande, D.R. (2012). A peculiar prevalence of p values just below .05. *Q. J. Exp. Psychol. (Hove).* 65: 2271–2279.

20. Perneger, T.V. and Combescure, C. (2017). The distribution of P-values in medical research articles suggested selective reporting associated with statistical significance. *J. Clin. Epidemiol.* 87: 70–77.

21. Leggett, N.C., Thomas, N.A., Loetscher, T. et al. (2013). The life of p: "just significant" results are on the rise. *Q. J. Exp. Psychol. (Hove).* 66: 2303–2309.

22. Ridley, J., Kolm, N., Freckelton, R.P. et al. (2007). An unexpected influence of widely used significance thresholds on the distribution of reported P-values. *J. Evol. Biol.* 20: 1082–1089.

23. Gadbury, G.L. and Allison, D.B. (2012). Inappropriate fiddling with statistical analyses to obtain a desirable p-value: tests to detect its presence in published literature. *PLoS One* https://doi.org/10.1371/journal.pone.0046363.

24. Schmucker, C., Schell, L.K., Portalupi, S. et al. (2014). Extent of non-publication in cohorts of studies approved by research eth-

ics committees or included in trial registries. *PLoS One* https://doi .org/10.1371/journal.pone.0114023.

25. Canestaro, W.J., Hendrix, N., Bansal, A. et al. (2017). Favorable and publicly funded studies are more likely to be published: a systematic review and meta-analysis. *J. Clin. Epidemiol.* 92: 58–68.

26. Dechartres, A., Atal, I., Riveros, C. et al. (2018). Association between publication characteristics and treatment effect estimates: a meta-epidemiologic study. *Ann. Intern. Med.* 169: 385–393.

27. Artino, A.R. Jr., Driessen, E.W., and Maggio, L.A. (2019). Ethical shades of gray: international frequency of scientific misconduct and questionable research practices in health professions education. *Acad. Med.* 94: 76–84.

28. Janke, S., Daumiller, M., and Rudert, S.C. (2019). Dark pathways to achievement in science: Researchers' achievement goals predict engagement in questionable research practices. *Soc. Psychol. Personal. Sci.* 10: 783–791.

29. John, L.K., Loewenstein, G., and Prelec, D. (2012). Measuring the prevalence of questionable research practices with incentives for truth telling. *Psychol. Sci.* 23: 524–532.

30. Lang, T. and Altman, D. (2014). Statistical analyses and methods in the published literature: the SAMPL guidelines. In: *Guidelines for Reporting Health Research: A User's Manual* (eds. D. Moher, D. Altman, K. Schulz, et al.), 265–274. Baltimore: Wiley.

31. Parsons, N.R., Price, C.L., Hiskens, R. et al. (2012). An evaluation of the quality of statistical design and analysis of published medical research: results from a systematic survey of general orthopaedic journals. *BMC Med. Res. Methodol.* https://doi .org/10.1186/1471-2288-12-60.

32. Prescott, R.J. and Civil, I. (2013). Lies, damn lies and statistics: errors and omission in papers submitted to INJURY 2010-2012. *Injury* 44: 6–11.

33. Nuijten, M.B., Hartgerink, C.H., van Assen, M.A. et al. (2016). The prevalence of statistical reporting errors in psychology (1985-2013). *Behav. Res. Methods* 48: 1205–1226.

34. Sacco, D.F., Bruton, S.V., and Brown, M. (2018). In defense of the questionable: defining the basis of research Scientists' engagement in questionable research practices. *J. Empir. Res. Hum. Res. Ethics* 13: 101–110.

35. Rubin, M. (2017). When does HARKing hurt? Identifying when different types of undisclosed post hoc hypothesizing harm scientific progress. *Rev. Gen. Psychol.* 21: 308–320.

36. Tijdink, J.K., Bouter, L.M., Veldkamp, C.L. et al. (2016). Personality traits are associated with research misbehavior in Dutch scientists: a cross-sectional study. *PLoS One* https://doi.org/10.1371/journal.pone.0163251.

37. Jennings, R.C. (2004). Data selection and responsible conduct: was Millikan a fraud? *Sci. Eng. Ethics* 10: 639–653.

38. Godecharle, S., Fieuws, S., Nemery, B. et al. (2018). Scientists still behaving badly? A survey within industry and universities. *Sci. Eng. Ethics* 24: 1697–1717.

39. Motulsky, H.J. (2015). Common misconceptions about data analysis and statistics. *Pharmacol. Res. Perspect.* 3: 200–205.

40. Austin, P.C., Mamdani, M.M., Juurlink, D.N. et al. (2006). Testing multiple statistical hypotheses resulted in spurious associations: a study of astrological signs and health. *J. Clin. Epidemiol.* 59: 964–969.

41. Li, G., Taljaard, M., Van den Heuvel, E.R. et al. (2017). An introduction to multiplicity issues in clinical trials: the what, why, when and how. *Int. J. Epidemiol.* 46: 746–755.

42. Vickerstaff, V., Ambler, G., King, M. et al. (2015). Are multiple primary outcomes analysed appropriately in randomised controlled trials? A review. *Contemp. Clin. Trials* 45: 8–12.

43. Tyler, K.M., Normand, S.L., and Horton, N.J. (2011). The use and abuse of multiple outcomes in randomized controlled depression trials. *Contemp. Clin. Trials* 32: 299–304.

44. Dwan, K., Gamble, C., Williamson, P.R. et al. (2013). Systematic review of the empirical evidence of study publication bias and outcome reporting bias – an updated review. *PLoS One* https://doi.org/10.1371/journal.pone.0066844.

45. Li, G., Abbade, L.P.F., Nwosu, I. et al. (2018). A systematic review of comparisons between protocols or registrations and full reports in primary biomedical research. *BMC Med. Res. Methodol.* https://doi.org/10.1186/s12874-017-0465-7.

46. Alosh, M., Bretz, F., and Huque, M. (2014). Advanced multiplicity adjustment methods in clinical trials. *Stat. Med.* 33: 693–713.

47. Wason, J.M., Stecher, L., and Mander, A.P. (2014). Correcting for multiple-testing in multi-arm trials: is it necessary and is it done? *Trials* https://doi.org/10.1186/1745-6215-15-364.

48. Kasenda, B., Schandelmaier, S., Sun, X. et al. (2014). Subgroup analyses in randomised controlled trials: cohort study on trial protocols and journal publications. *BMJ* https://doi.org/10.1136/bmj.g4539.

49. Sun, X., Briel, M., Busse, J.W. et al. (2012). Credibility of claims of subgroup effects in randomised controlled trials: systematic review. *BMJ* https://doi.org/10.1136/bmj.l4898.

50. Wallach, J.D., Sullivan, P.G., Trepanowski, J.F. et al. (2017). Evaluation of evidence of statistical support and corroboration of subgroup claims in randomized clinical trials. *JAMA Intern. Med.* 177: 554–560.

51. Sun, X., Ioannidis, J.P., Agoritsas, T. et al. (2014). How to use a subgroup analysis: users' guide to the medical literature. *JAMA* 311: 405–411.

52. Burke, J.F., Sussman, J.B., Kent, D.M. et al. (2015). Three simple rules to ensure reasonably credible subgroup analyses. *BMJ* https://doi.org/10.1136/bmj.h5651.

53. Sun, X., Briel, M., Walter, S.D. et al. (2010). Is a subgroup effect believable? Updating criteria to evaluate the credibility of subgroup analyses. *BMJ* https://doi.org/10.1136/bmj.c117.

54. Fan, J., Song, F., and Bachmann, M.O. (2018). Justification and reporting of subgroup analyses were lacking or inadequate in randomised controlled trials. *J. Clin. Epidemiol.* 108: 17–25.

55. Sleight, P. (2000). Debate: subgroup analyses in clinical trials: fun to look at – but don't believe them! *Curr. Control Trials Cardiovasc. Med.* 1: 25–27.

56. Yu, L.M., Chan, A.W., Hopewell, S. et al. (2010). Reporting on covariate adjustment in randomised controlled trials before and after revision of the 2001 CONSORT statement: a literature review. *Trials* https://doi.org/10.1186/1745-6215-11-59.

57. Kahan, B.C., Jairath, V., Dore, C.J. et al. (2014). The risks and rewards of covariate adjustment in randomized trials: an assessment of 12 outcomes from 8 studies. *Trials* https://doi.org/10.1186/1745-6215-15-139.

58. Raab, G.M., Day, S., and Sales, J. (2000). How to select covariates to include in the analysis of a clinical trial. *Control. Clin. Trials* 21: 330–342.

59. Schulz, K.F., Altman, D.G., and Moher, D. (2010). CONSORT 2010 statement: updated guidelines for reporting parallel group randomised trials. *BMJ* https://doi.org/10.1136/bmj.f4313.

60. Lee, P.H. (2016). Covariate adjustments in randomized controlled trials increased study power and reduced biasedness of effect size estimation. *J. Clin. Epidemiol.* 76: 137–146.

61. Saquib, N., Saquib, J., and Ioannidis, J.P. (2013). Practices and impact of primary outcome adjustment in randomized controlled trials: meta-epidemiologic study. *BMJ* https://doi.org/10.1136/bmj.f4313.

62. Gamble, C., Krishan, A., Stocken, D. et al. (2017). Guidelines for the content of statistical analysis plans in clinical trials. *JAMA* 318: 2337–2343.

63. Greenberg, L., Jairath, V., Pearse, R. et al. (2018). Pre-specification of statistical analysis approaches in published clinical trial protocols was inadequate. *J. Clin. Epidemiol.* 101: 53–60.

64. Dwan, K., Altman, D.G., Clarke, M. et al. (2014). Evidence for the selective reporting of analyses and discrepancies in clinical trials: a systematic review of cohort studies of clinical trials. *PLoS Med.* https://doi.org/10.1371/journal.pmed.1001666.

65. Fanelli, D. (2012). Negative results are disappearing from most disciplines and countries. *Scientometrics* 90: 891–904.

66. Monsarrat, P. and Vergnes, J.N. (2018). The intriguing evolution of effect sizes in biomedical research over time: smaller but more often statistically significant. *GigaScience* https://doi.org/10.1093/gigascience/gix121.

67. Wang, M.Q., Yan, A.F., and Katz, R.V. (2018). Researcher requests for inappropriate analysis and reporting: a U.S. survey of consulting biostatisticians. *Ann. Intern. Med.* 169: 554–558.

68. Wang, M.Q., Fan, A.Y., and Katz, R.V. (2019). Bioethical issues in biostatistical consulting study: additional findings and concerns. *JDR Clin. Trans. Res.* 4: 271–275.

69. Wicherts, J.M., Veldkamp, C.L., Augusteijn, H.E. et al. (2016). Degrees of freedom in planning, running, analyzing, and reporting psychological studies: a checklist to avoid p-hacking. *Front. Psychol.* https://doi.org/10.3389/fpsyg.2016.01832.

70. Forstmeier, W., Wagenmakers, E.J., and Parker, T.H. (2017). Detecting and avoiding likely false-positive findings – a practical guide. *Biol. Rev. Camb. Philos. Soc.* 92: 1941–1968.

71. Ebrahim, S., Sohani, Z.N., Montoya, L. et al. (2014). Reanalyses of randomized clinical trial data. *JAMA* 312: 1024–1032.

72. Colquhoun, D. (2014). An investigation of the false discovery rate and the misinterpretation of p-values. *R. Soc. Open Sci.* https://doi .org/10.1098/rsos.140216.

CHAPTER 5

Systematic Reviews and Meta-Analysis

INTRODUCTION

Review papers should provide convenient summaries of all relevant clinical trials. Although such summaries are a long-standing feature of the medical literature, a seminal paper by Cynthia Mulrow in 1987 [1] raised serious concerns about the quality of the review process. She found that many reviews were based on somewhat haphazard literature searches, and only a few evaluated the methodological quality of the studies that they identified. These weaknesses threaten the validity of the review findings. Since then, several research groups have developed more systematic approaches to identify all the relevant studies and to appraise their quality [2]. This led to a set of rigorous methods to identify and synthesise all the evidence on the effectiveness of a treatment. Detailed guidance on the conduct of systematic reviews has been produced by several

Evidence in Medicine: The Common Flaws, Why They Occur and How to Prevent Them, First Edition. Iain K Crombie.
© 2021 John Wiley & Sons Ltd. Published 2021 by John Wiley & Sons Ltd.

organisations including the Cochrane Collaboration [3], the US Institute of Medicine [4] and the Centre for Reviews and Dissemination [5].

Meta-Analysis

Many clinical trials consist of small numbers of patients [6], so their estimates of treatment effects can be affected by the play of chance. This means that the individual studies will sometimes overestimate treatment benefits, and other times will underestimate them. To overcome this problem, the results of individual trials of a treatment can be combined to provide a more precise estimate of the benefit of a treatment. The term meta-analysis refers to the statistical methods used to combine the findings from individual trials into a single summary estimate of treatment benefit [7]. It was first proposed by Glass in 1976, as a way of combining studies in education research [8]. He was concerned about 'pedestrian reviewing where verbal synopses of studies are strung out in dizzying lists'. Glass found that the methodologies that were then used to combine studies were 'too weak for the complexity of the problem', and proposed a more robust method for combining the effects from individual studies. His work stimulated efforts to develop powerful statistical methods to pool effect sizes across trials. These methods provide combined estimates of treatment effects that have high precision (i.e. low uncertainty) [9].

Aims of the Chapter

Despite the readily accessible guidance on systematic reviews, there is widespread concern that many are poorly conducted [10–13]. In addition, many meta-analyses provide inadequate descriptions of the methods used [14]. This chapter assesses the evidence for the main pitfalls and biases of systematic reviews and meta-analysis. It does so by exploring four key stages of systematic reviews: 1) the identification of relevant trials, 2) extraction of key data items from the trials, 3) assessment of the quality of the trials and 4) pooling trials to provide summary estimates.

IDENTIFYING RELEVANT TRIALS

The great strength of systematic reviews is that they can provide unbiased estimates of treatment effect because they combine data from all the trials of specific treatments. Three problems threaten this benefit: unpublished trials, inadequate literature searches and the process of screening for relevant trials.

Unpublished Studies

Many trials are completed but not published in medical journals. These studies are often not included in systematic reviews, leading to biased estimates of treatment benefit. An example of this is the drug Reboxetine, which early systematic reviews had found to be effective and safe [15]. A more careful review in 2010 established that nearly three quarters (74%) of the patient data on this drug had not been published. When this new material was included in a systematic review, it showed that Reboxetine was an 'ineffective and potentially harmful antidepressant' [15]. Similarly systematic reviews had concluded that the drug Tamiflu, which was widely used during the 2009 swine flu pandemic, reduced hospitalisations and complications of influenza [16]. Subsequent investigation showed that many trials were not published or were selectively published [17]. Analysis of all the data revealed that the drug had no significant effect on either hospitalisations or serious complications of flu, but did cause adverse effects such as nausea and vomiting and renal and psychiatric problems [18].

These examples raise the question of how often trials are not published. To explore this, researchers have identified all the studies listed in several locations: international trial registries, such as http://Clinicaltrials.gov; data held by research funders; or trials approved by research ethics committees. The resulting lists are then compared with trials that were subsequently published (i.e. found after searching bibliographic databases). An overview of 39 such studies confirmed that there is substantial non-publication [19]. It found that, on average, about one half of the trials listed on the registry databases and ethical committee records were not published.

Bias from Unpublished Studies

Comparisons of unpublished and published studies consistently show that published studies are more likely to have significant findings and larger effect sizes than unpublished ones [19–22]. The important question concerns the extent to which unpublished studies could distort estimates of treatment benefit. This has been explored by comparing the effect sizes when these studies are excluded and included. One early study reanalysed 42 meta-analyses [23] and found that the addition of unpublished data sometimes increased the estimated effect sizes, but could also lead to decreased estimates. Large changes in effect size only occurred when a substantial proportion of trial data was unpublished. Similar findings have been reported in more recent studies [24–26]. It seems that inclusion of unpublished trials sometimes produces a small to modest decrease in estimated treatment benefit, or it can it increase the effect size. For an individual systematic review, in the absence of extensive checking, it is difficult to know what difference unpublished studies might make.

Given these concerns, systematic reviewers are strongly advised to explore whether publication bias could have occurred [3–5]. Several simple statistical techniques have been developed to assist this evaluation [27, 28]. Overviews of sets of systematic reviews have shown that most systematic reviews do not test for publication bias: in a random sample of 300 systematic reviews published in February 2014, only 31% did so [14]. The frequency of this testing may vary across specialties, as 43% of systematic reviews in anaesthesiology assessed publication bias [29], but only 28% did so in oncology [30], 22% in dermatology [31] and 0% in burns care [32]. However in high quality journals, 69% of reviews reported an evaluation of publication bias [33]. Although publication bias can be important, this issue is commonly not investigated with sufficient vigour.

Adequacy of the Sources Searched

Electronic databases, such as MEDLINE, EMBASE, CENTRAL, CINAHL and LILACS contain listings of trials published in medical and health professional journals [34]. As they differ somewhat in coverage, it is recommended that at least three databases should be searched [35]. Searching of only one database was once common practice, but more recent systematic reviews now search an average of 3.7 databases [36]. However many reviews still only search one or two databases. The Cochrane Handbook for Systematic Reviews strongly recommends (on pp. 71 and 75) [3] that several databases should be searched.

International registries of clinical trials, such as http://clinicaltrials.gov, http://ISRCTN.com and the International Clinical Trials Registry Platform, can be used to identify unpublished trials. The Cochrane Handbook [3] (on p. 67) strongly recommends such searches. However many systematic reviews do not access them: the proportions that do ranged from 18% to 48% in different overviews [25, 37, 38]. An evaluation of 95 systematic reviews that did not search trial registries found that the more extensive search often identified additional trials [25]. It concluded that 'trial registers are an important source of additional RCTs'.

The other source to search is the grey literature: this comprises conference papers, theses, book chapters and other reports that are not published in conventional academic journals [39, 40]. Searching these sources is recommended [41], but is considered less important than electronic databases and trials registries [3]. Several studies have shown that searching this literature yields few additional trials, and that these often have little impact on estimates of treatment benefit [24, 26]. The current challenge is 'to identify which reviews may benefit most from including unpublished or grey data' [26].

In summary the diversity of sources searched, particularly of databases and trial registries, is commonly inadequate [42]. Failing to include all relevant trials in a review could bias the estimated treatment benefit [43, 44].

Problems with the Search Strategies

To ensure all relevant trials are identified, systematic reviews should employ comprehensive search strategies. Searches of electronic databases combine search terms in a logical sequence to ensure that all potentially relevant studies are identified. Evaluating the quality of the strategies is difficult because only a few systematic reviews publish their full search strategies: overview studies found the proportion doing so ranged from 10.5% to 24% [45–47]. When search strategies are stated, deficiencies that would limit the coverage of the search occur in 53%–78% of systematic reviews [48, 49].

The important question is how many papers are unknowingly omitted from systematic reviews. One group investigated this by identifying all the trials in a specific field, advanced non-small cell lung cancer. They found that systematic reviews only identified between 45% and 70% of the relevant trials [50]. A similar study in traumatic brain injury found that only 65% of systematic reviews included all the relevant trials [13]. It seems likely that search strategies often fail to identify all the relevant studies, which could lead to biased estimates of treatment effect.

Screening for Relevant Trials

Search strategies usually identify thousands of papers which need to be screened to identify those that are likely to be relevant. To achieve this, detailed eligibility criteria for inclusion should be stated. These usually cover the years of publication, the types of patients studied, the treatment given, the length of follow-up and the outcome measures used. Not all systematic reviews report these details, with estimates of the proportions doing so ranging from 50% to 90% [51–53].

Screening is a two stage process, involving an examination of the titles and abstracts of potentially relevant studies, then obtaining full copies of the most likely candidates to identify the trials for inclusion. This process is subjective, so the work should be conducted by two reviewers [54]. Careful examination has shown that if conducted by a single person, many relevant studies are missed [54, 55]. Several evaluations of this process found that only about one half of systematic reviews use two reviewers to identify studies for inclusion [51–53]. Another problem is that the eligibility criteria are not always followed: an overview of systematic reviews for irritable bowel showed that up to 29% of the trials included in reviews were ineligible according to the stated inclusion criteria [56]. The process of selecting trials for inclusion in systematic reviews could be improved.

EXTRACTING TRIAL DATA

The most important data items for a systematic review are the outcome measures collected at baseline and follow-up, together with their standard deviations, and the numbers of patients in the trials. Assessment of how well these are extracted provides a guide to the quality of the data extraction process. Research has shown that there are often errors in this process.

Incorrect Data

Errors are frequently made in the extraction of the outcome data [57]. These come in two varieties. Some are errors due to misinterpretation, such as mistaking a median for a mean, or a standard error for a standard deviation [58]. More common are simple typographical errors that can affect the number of participants, the outcomes of trials (such as the number of events) and the standard deviations [58–60]. The impact of these errors on the estimate of treatment effect can be assessed by repeating the meta-analysis with corrected data. An overview of such studies found that the errors had only a moderate effect on the estimated treatment benefit, but did not affect the reviews' conclusions [57].

Multiple Outcomes

Clinical trials usually report data on several outcomes: one overview of eye disease studies reported a median of five outcomes per trial [61], and for trials in HIV the median was eight [62]. Sometimes the total number of outcomes exceeds the number of trials that have been conducted: among 524 HIV trials there were 779 unique outcomes [62], and for the drug gabapentin, 21 trials reported 214 different outcomes [63]. This diversity is partly due to an outcome being measured by different instruments: among 104 trials of complex regional pain syndrome, 68 different outcome questionnaires were used to measure pain [64]. In addition, the data from identical instruments can presented in differing ways. They can be measured at several timepoints, scales from questionnaires can be presented as a mean score or a per cent exceeding a defined threshold, and scores can be presented as the outcome at follow-up or as the difference from baseline [65, 66]. This diversity of measuring was seen in an evaluation of 61 cardiac arrest trials [67]. Although survival was the most common outcome, it was assessed in 39 different ways. A consequence of the multiplicity of possible outcomes is that trials of a particular treatment often collect and present data on important outcomes in ways that mean the findings cannot be included in systematic reviews. This makes it more difficult to draw clear conclusions about effectiveness, and leads to wasted research [68].

Outcome Reporting Bias

The profusion of outcome measures creates a more serious problem: the process of selecting which outcomes to include could affect the result in a meta-analysis. Systematic reviews commonly present many fewer outcome measures than are reported in clinical trials [61, 62, 69]. Statistically significant findings are more likely to be included in a systematic review than non-significant ones [70]. Further Mayo-Wilson and colleagues have demonstrated that cherry picking the outcome from the large variety on offer could make an intervention appear either effective or ineffective [66]. At present, there is no clear evidence that selective inclusion of outcomes affects the estimates of treatment effect [71].

In theory the problem of outcome selection could be prevented if systematic reviews pre-specified their primary outcome in a published paper or in the PROSPERO international registry of protocols of reviews [72]. In practice there are often differences between the published primary outcome and the registered one, with stated primary outcomes being omitted or downgraded to secondary outcomes and new outcomes added [73]. These changes are common, with estimates of discrepancies in outcomes ranging from 22% to 45% of systematic reviews [73–76]. Well-intentioned, but motivated, selection of outcomes could lead to bias in the estimates of treatment benefit.

Adverse Events

Systematic reviews should provide good estimates of the frequency of adverse events [77]. Instead, they often fail to report the harms data from completed trials [78, 79]. For example, one third of 78 reviews in gastroenterology made no mention of harms in the body of the paper, and only 8% presented numerical data on harms in the abstract [80]. These data led the authors to conclude that 'the reporting of harms. . . is largely inadequate', a conclusion that was also drawn by another survey of systematic reviews [81]. The interpretation of adverse events can also be poor; Mahady and colleagues highlighted one systematic review that recognised that adverse events were not well reported but concluded that 'adverse events are minimal and the risk benefit ratio is good' [80].

Poor reporting may occur because most reviews do not include an assessment of harms as an outcome measure [80]; possibly a beneficial outcome is considered more interesting than a harmful one. Even when an adverse event was listed as an outcome measure, most reviews reported the data incompletely and many did not report it at all [78]. The extent of this problem has led to new guidance for the reporting of harms in systematic reviews [82]. Reliable evidence on harms will only become available when this guidance is routinely followed.

THE QUALITY OF PRIMARY TRIALS

The value of systematic reviews depends on the quality of the clinical trials that they analyse. The Cochrane Handbook of Systematic Reviews [3] strongly encourages (p. 187) that the quality of the primary trials be assessed using a risk of bias tool. Two studies covering several thousand systematic reviews found that about 70% assessed the risk of bias of the included studies [14, 52]. This figure may conceal substantial variation across medical specialties. In anaesthesia journals 84% of reviews assessed the quality of trials [83] but only 33% of reviews in burns care [32].

Taking Quality into Account

Systematic reviews that assess quality often find that the quality of many of the included trials is poor, placing them at high risk of bias [83, 84]. Most systematic reviews conduct a formal risk of bias assessment [11, 12, 14, 85], although there are exceptions to this [32, 86]. The important question is whether the quality of the trials is taken into account during the analysis and interpretation of the findings, with risk of bias reducing the strength of the conclusions [3] (pp. 190–192). Although most reviews measure the quality of included trials, they do not use these assessments to explore the impact of bias [11, 14, 85]. For example, they could calculate the pooled effect size with all the trials included, then do this again for only the high quality trials. If the estimates are markedly different, the poor quality trials are likely to be biased. In some cases there are simply too few high quality trials to justify the exploratory analyses [84]. The poor quality of many trials, and the bias they may introduce and are an unresolved issues for systematic reviews.

POOLING EFFECT SIZES ACROSS TRIALS

Meta-analyses use statistical methods to pool the effect sizes from individual trials to provide an overall average for all trials. The process involves assigning a weight to each trial. The weight depends on a measure of the variance of the effect size (roughly corresponding to the sample size), so that larger trials have a bigger effect on the overall average than small ones.

There are two formal approaches for estimating the average effect size: fixed effects models and random effects models [87]. The simpler one is the fixed effects model. It assumes that all the trials in the systematic review provide estimates of a single, but unknown, treatment effect: technically they are all sampling from the same population. In contrast the random effects model assumes that the individual trials can come from different populations and that they provide estimates of (slightly) different effect sizes.

Heterogeneity

The trials included in a systematic review may vary in factors such as the characteristics of the patients included (e.g. age or disease severity), the way the treatment was delivered or in the length of follow-up. Studies can also differ in the extent to which they are at risk of bias from factors such as allocation concealment and blinding of outcome assessment. If these factors varied markedly across trials, this would create real differences in the effect sizes across the trials included in a systematic review. The consequence is heterogeneity; this occurs when the treatment effects differ more than would be expected from the play of chance alone.

When the included trials clearly differ in their clinical characteristics and methodological quality, one option is to present the data from the trials (effect size and standard deviation) without conducting a meta-analysis [88]. The Cochrane Handbook of Systematic Reviews [3] (p. 232) recommends careful tabulation of the key elements of the trials to assist in this assessment. However, if there is broad similarity across the trials, researchers can use fixed effects models or random effects models to synthesise the data. If the observed heterogeneity is small, fixed effects models could be used, if it is large random effects might be the better choice.

Heterogeneity is most commonly measured by the I-squared statistic, I^2. This ranges from 0% to 100% and measures the proportion of the variation in treatment effects that is due to real differences between studies (rather than to the play of chance). Some authors suggest that random effects models should be used when $I^2 \geq 25\%$ [89], although others put the level at $I^2 \geq 50\%$ [90]. The Cochrane Handbook of Systematic Reviews [3] (p. 259) provides 'a rough guide to the interpretation' of I^2:

- 0%–40%: might not be important
- 30%–60%: may represent moderate heterogeneity
- 50%–90%: may represent substantial heterogeneity
- 75%–100%: considerable heterogeneity

Current practice on when to use fixed effects and random effects models is highly varied. A survey of 110 published meta-analyses found that the threshold used to identify substantial heterogeneity ranged from 25% to 75%, with 43% using $I^2 \geq 50\%$ [91]. A review of 72 systematic reviews found that some studies used fixed effects models with $I^2 \geq 60\%$, and many with $I^2 \leq 30\%$ used random effects models [92]. Another study found that 48% of systematic reviews that specified how they would use I^2 (or a similar measure) to select fixed or random effects models, did not follow their proposed plan [93]. It is likely that some meta-analyses may be using inappropriate methods for pooling data.

Exploring Heterogeneity

When there is evidence of heterogeneity, statistical methods can be used to identify the factors (participants, study methods and sources of bias) that are causing it [94, 95]. (This involves fitting regression models to assess the extent to which these factors can explain (reduce) heterogeneity.) In practice many meta-analyses do not investigate the causes of heterogeneity. One study of reviews in the field of pregnancy and childbirth found that 65% of the reviews with high heterogeneity did not explore it [93]. In a more recent study of Cochrane reviews, 98% planned to explore heterogeneity and 63% did so. None assessed the plausibility or importance of these explanatory factors [96]. As Chess and Gagnier commented 'there is room for improvement in assessing clinical heterogeneity' [97].

OTHER METHODOLOGICAL ISSUES

Missing Outcome Data

Most clinical trials have some missing outcome data that could bias the estimate of treatment effect, leading in turn to bias in the summary estimates of effectiveness of meta-analyses [98]. One overview study found that, although many systematic reviews reported missing data in the trials they included, only 19% had plans to deal with this in their analyses [99]. A separate study found that Cochrane reviews were more likely to have a plan for handling missing data (41%) than non-Cochrane reviews (9%) [100].

The recommended approach to handling missing data in meta-analysis is to calculate effect sizes using all the available data, then conduct sensitivity analyses in which different assumptions are made about the nature of the missing data (e.g. those missing are the same on average as those not missing, or they are biased to a small or to a large extent) [98]. This approach sheds light on the extent to which the missing data could affect the estimate of effectiveness. Overview studies have found that less than 20% of meta-analyses described methods for sensitivity analyses, and fewer still conducted them [99–101]. Missing outcome data, a potential source of bias, is often poorly dealt with in meta-analyses.

The Sparse Data Problem

Many systematic reviews include only small numbers of trials, with estimates of the median number ranging between three and seven [102–104]. Most of the trials comprise less than 100 participants [6, 102], so that most systematic reviews consist entirely of small underpowered trials [105]. (Underpowered means unlikely to detect a clinically worthwhile benefit as being statistically significant.) This helps explain why about one half of systematic reviews are unable to identify whether treatments are effective or not: the pooled sample sizes are not large enough to provide useful evidence [106, 107]. Other factors contributing to inconclusive reviews are high heterogeneity and poor quality of the included trials [107, 108]. Although systematic reviews should provide a reliable (high precision) estimate of treatment benefit, many do not. Instead, they often conclude that more large, high quality trials are needed [106–108]; despite the many thousands of trials conducted each year, sparse data limit the evidence on effectiveness.

Conflicting Findings

In general, different meta-analyses on a specific treatment should come to similar conclusions. However sometimes meta-analyses have discordant findings [109]. This can occur when overlapping sets of trials are included in the meta-analyses [110]. The combination of including differing sets of trials, which used different outcome measures and analytic methods, explained discrepant findings in studies of vitamin D9 [111]. Methodological errors (incorrect application of eligibility criteria and problems with data extraction and analysis) can also lead to conflicting findings: these were identified as the reason for differing conclusions among systematic reviews of probiotics [112].

Conflict in meta-analyses of progestogens in pregnancy identified a different cause. Across 29 reviews, 19 concluded the drugs were effective, 1 advised caution and 7 stated that the drugs were ineffective [113]. In an attempt to resolve the conflict, a further analysis focused on those trials that had pre-registered their primary outcomes. It found no effect of the drugs. The researchers suggested that the discrepancy between systematic reviews could be due to 'silently switched outcomes' in the unregistered trials [113].

The quality and completeness of reporting data on harms provide another possible cause of conflict between systematic reviews. Systematic reviews of thrombolytic therapy for pulmonary embolism were broadly in agreement on the benefits of treatment but had different findings on harms, leading to disputes about the net benefit of treatment [114].

The occurrence of systematic reviews with conflicting findings highlights the impact of the methods used on the conclusions drawn. When conflicting findings occur, a detailed examination of the methods of the reviews can help unravel the causes. In general, for an individual systematic review, the methods should be carefully reviewed to clarify their likely impact on the findings.

Wasted and Redundant Systematic Reviews

The number of published systematic reviews has increased dramatically since the 1980s [109], but many provide little or no additional evidence [115]. Much of this waste results from poor quality methods, with failings in the search strategies, data extraction, assessment of risk of bias, and lack of checking for publication bias [14], as well as switching of outcome measures [73].

Waste also occurs when several meta-analyses are conducted on nearly identical sets of trials. For example 57 meta-analyses of non-vitamin K oral anticoagulants in atrial fibrillation collated data from only 14 clinical trials, with substantial overlap between reviews [116]. Riaz and colleagues documented a further 10 topics with overlapping and redundant systematic reviews. The most extreme case was of a treatment for stroke, in which 17 reviews were conducted on three trials; 13 of these reviews were conducted over a 6 month period [117]. Another study found considerable overlap in reviews of statins for atrial fibrillation after surgery [118]. As Ioannidis concluded, 'there is a massive production of unnecessary, misleading and conflicted systematic reviews and meta-analyses' [109].

CONCLUSIONS

Systematic reviews should provide the best evidence on the effectiveness of treatments. In theory, they identify all the relevant randomised controlled trials and summarise their findings to provide 'a transparent outline of the balance between the benefits and harms of healthcare behaviour and interventions' [77]. Other advantages include greater precision in the estimate of treatment effect and an evaluation of potential sources of bias.

In practice many, some say most, of the systematic reviews are of poor quality and are likely to lead to misleading or unhelpful conclusions [77]. The number of systematic reviews and meta-analyses published each year has increased exponentially from 435 in 1995 to 20,774 in 2017 [119]. The number of systematic reviews that are published each year (20,774) is similar to the number of clinical trials being published (22,560) [119]. Ioannidis and colleagues have estimated that only 3% of reviews were well conducted and clinically useful [109].

This chapter has outlined deficiencies in the four key stages of systematic reviews: searching for trials, extracting the data, assessing the quality of the trials and pooling estimates across trials. Problems are common, although each deficiency has only a modest influence on the estimated treatment effects. However, if several flaws occur together, the cumulative effect could be large. One example for this comes from an assessment of trials on the treatment of depression [120]. This found that each of the factors publication bias, outcome selection bias, and spin and citation bias resulted in trials with negative findings being excluded from the evidence base. However these biases had an additive impact so that 'the effects of different biases accumulate to hide nonsignificant results from view' [120]. A different example is from severe traumatic brain injury, where the combination of lack of completeness (i.e. some relevant trials omitted) and poor methodological quality of the systematic reviews contributed to 'potentially unreliable evidence underpinning practice' [13]. As the Cochrane Handbook points out (on p. 241), meta-analyses 'have the potential to mislead seriously, particularly if specific study designs, within-study biases, variations across studies, and reporting biases are not carefully considered' [3].

In addition to their own methodological problems, systematic reviews are vulnerable to the quality of the trials they include. Poor quality trials and outcome reporting bias can distort the raw data that systematic reviews use. The quality of the included trials is frequently assessed by reviews, but only a minority takes quality into account when analysing the data and interpreting the findings. The systematic review may otherwise be of high quality, but if the trials are methodologically weak, the estimates of treatment effects could be biased.

In summary, systematic reviews have great potential, but often come with many flaws. Some 20 years ago a commentator posed the question, 'Systematic reviews of published evidence: miracles or minefields?' [121]. A more recent assessment of their contribution sounded a similarly cautious note 'Are systematic reviews and meta-analyses still useful research? We are not sure' [77]. Many of the threats to the validity of systematic reviews could be overcome, or at least ameliorated, by careful design and execution [77]. Until the issues of quality are resolved, systematic reviews should be assumed to be flawed, until a detailed examination has proven otherwise.

REFERENCES

1. Mulrow, C.D. (1987). The medical review article: state of the science. *Ann. Intern. Med.* 106: 485–488.
2. Chalmers, I., Hedges, L.V., and Cooper, H. (2002). A brief history of research synthesis. *Eval. Health Prof.* 25: 12–37.
3. Higgins, J., Thomas, J., Chandler, J. et al. (eds.) (2019). *Cochrane Handbook for Systematic Reviews of Interventions*, 2e. Chichester: Wiley.
4. Eden, J., Levit, L., Berg, A. et al. (eds.) (2011). *Finding What Works in Health Care: Standards for Systematic Reviews*. Washington: National Academies Press.
5. CRD (2009). *Systematic Reviews*. York: University of York.
6. Califf, R.M., Zarin, D.A., Kramer, J.M. et al. (2012). Characteristics of clinical trials registered in ClinicalTrials.gov, 2007–2010. *JAMA* 307: 1838–1847.
7. Gurevitch, J., Koricheva, J., Nakagawa, S. et al. (2018). Meta-analysis and the science of research synthesis. *Nature* 555: 175–182.
8. Glass, G.V. (1976). Primary, secondary, and meta-analysis of research. *Educ. Res.* 5: 3–8.
9. Borenstein, M., Hedges, L.V., Higgins, J.P.T. et al. (2009). *Introduction to Meta-Analysis*. Chichester: Wiley.
10. Roush, G.C., Amante, B., Singh, T. et al. (2016). Quality of meta-analyses for randomized trials in the field of hypertension: a systematic review. *J. Hypertens.* 34: 2305–2317.
11. Koster, T.M., Wetterslev, J., Gluud, C. et al. (2018). Systematic overview and critical appraisal of meta-analyses of interventions in intensive care medicine. *Acta Anaesthesiol. Scand.* https://doi.org/10.1111/aas.13147.
12. Evaniew, N., van der Watt, L., Bhandari, M. et al. (2015). Strategies to improve the credibility of meta-analyses in spine surgery: a systematic survey. *Spine J.* 15: 2066–2076.
13. Synnot, A., Bragge, P., Lunny, C. et al. (2018). The currency, completeness and quality of systematic reviews of acute management of

moderate to severe traumatic brain injury: a comprehensive evidence map. *PLoS One* https://doi.org/10.1371/journal.pone.0198676.

14. Page, M.J., Shamseer, L., Altman, D.G. et al. (2016). Epidemiology and reporting characteristics of systematic reviews of biomedical research: a cross-sectional study. *PLoS Med.* https://doi.org/10.1371/journal.pmed.1002028.

15. Eyding, D., Lelgemann, M., Grouven, U. et al. (2010). Reboxetine for acute treatment of major depression: systematic review and meta-analysis of published and unpublished placebo and selective serotonin reuptake inhibitor controlled trials. *BMJ* https://doi.org/10.1136/bmj.c4737.

16. Kaiser, L., Wat, C., Mills, T. et al. (2003). Impact of oseltamivir treatment on influenza-related lower respiratory tract complications and hospitalizations. *Arch. Intern. Med.* 163: 1667–1672.

17. Doshi, P. (2009). Neuraminidase inhibitors – the story behind the Cochrane review. *BMJ* https://doi.org/10.1136/bmj.b5164.

18. Jefferson, T., Jones, M.A., Doshi, P. et al. (2014). Neuraminidase inhibitors for preventing and treating influenza in healthy adults and children. *Cochrane Database Syst. Rev.* https://doi.org/10.1002/14651858.CD008965.pub4.

19. Schmucker, C., Schell, L.K., Portalupi, S. et al. (2014). Extent of non-publication in cohorts of studies approved by research ethics committees or included in trial registries. *PLoS One* https://doi.org/10.1371/journal.pone.0114023.

20. Canestaro, W.J., Hendrix, N., Bansal, A. et al. (2017). Favorable and publicly funded studies are more likely to be published: a systematic review and meta-analysis. *J. Clin. Epidemiol.* 92: 58–68.

21. Song, S.Y., Koo, D.H., Jung, S.Y. et al. (2017). The significance of the trial outcome was associated with publication rate and time to publication. *J. Clin. Epidemiol.* 84: 78–84.

22. Dechartres, A., Atal, I., Riveros, C. et al. (2018). Association between publication characteristics and treatment effect estimates: a meta-epidemiologic study. *Ann. Intern. Med.* 169: 385–393.

23. Hart, B., Lundh, A., and Bero, L. (2012). Effect of reporting bias on meta-analyses of drug trials: reanalysis of meta-analyses. *BMJ* https://doi.org/10.1136/bmj.d7202.

24. Hartling, L., Featherstone, R., Nuspl, M. et al. (2017). Grey literature in systematic reviews: a cross-sectional study of the contribution of non-English reports, unpublished studies and dissertations to the results of meta-analyses in child-relevant reviews. *BMC Med. Res. Methodol.* https://doi.org/10.1186/s12874-017-0347-z.

25. Baudard, M., Yavchitz, A., Ravaud, P. et al. (2017). Impact of searching clinical trial registries in systematic reviews of pharmaceutical treatments: methodological systematic review and reanalysis of meta-analyses. *BMJ* https://doi.org/10.1136/bmj.d561.

26. Schmucker, C.M., Blumle, A., Schell, L.K. et al. (2017). Systematic review finds that study data not published in full text articles have unclear impact on meta-analyses results in medical research. *PLoS One* https://doi.org/10.1371/journal.pone.0176210.

27. Peters, J.L., Sutton, A.J., Jones, D.R. et al. (2008). Contour-enhanced meta-analysis funnel plots help distinguish publication bias from other causes of asymmetry. *J. Clin. Epidemiol.* 61: 991–996.

28. Duval, S. and Tweedie, R. (2000). Trim and fill: a simple funnel-plot-based method of testing and adjusting for publication bias in meta-analysis. *Biometrics* 56: 455–463.

29. Hedin, R.J., Umberham, B.A., Detweiler, B.N. et al. (2016). Publication bias and nonreporting found in majority of systematic reviews and meta-analyses in anesthesiology journals. *Anesth. Analg.* 123: 1018–1025.

30. Herrmann, D., Sinnett, P., Holmes, J. et al. (2017). Statistical controversies in clinical research: publication bias evaluations are not routinely conducted in clinical oncology systematic reviews. *Ann. Oncol.* 28: 931–937.

31. Atakpo, P. and Vassar, M. (2016). Publication bias in dermatology systematic reviews and meta-analyses. *J. Dermatol. Sci.* 82: 69–74.

32. Campbell, J.M., Kavanagh, S., Kurmis, R. et al. (2017). Systematic reviews in burns care: poor quality and getting worse. *J. Burn Care Res.* 38: e552–e567.

33. Onishi, A. and Furukawa, T.A. (2014). Publication bias is underreported in systematic reviews published in high-impact-factor journals: metaepidemiologic study. *J. Clin. Epidemiol.* 67: 1320–1326.

34. Betran, A.P., Say, L., Gulmezoglu, A.M. et al. (2005). Effectiveness of different databases in identifying studies for systematic

reviews: experience from the WHO systematic review of maternal morbidity and mortality. *BMC Med. Res. Methodol.* https://doi.org/10.1186/1471-2288-5-6.

35. Aagaard, T., Lund, H., and Juhl, C. (2016). Optimizing literature search in systematic reviews – are MEDLINE, EMBASE and CENTRAL enough for identifying effect studies within the area of musculoskeletal disorders? *BMC Med. Res. Methodol.* https://doi.org/10.1186/s12874-016-0264-6.

36. Lam, M.T. and McDiarmid, M. (2016). Increasing number of databases searched in systematic reviews and meta-analyses between 1994 and 2014. *J. Med. Libr. Assoc.* 104: 284–289.

37. Bibens, M.E., Chong, A.B., and Vassar, M. (2016). Utilization of clinical trials registries in obstetrics and gynecology systematic reviews. *Obstet. Gynecol.* 127: 248–253.

38. Jones, C.W., Keil, L.G., Weaver, M.A. et al. (2014). Clinical trials registries are under-utilized in the conduct of systematic reviews: a cross-sectional analysis. *Syst. Rev.* https://doi.org/10.1186/2046-4053-3-126.

39. Mahood, Q., Van Eerd, D., and Irvin, E. (2014). Searching for grey literature for systematic reviews: challenges and benefits. *Res. Synth. Methods* 5: 221–234.

40. Paez, A. (2017). Gray literature: an important resource in systematic reviews. *J. Evid. Based Med.* 10: 233–240.

41. Cooper, C., Booth, A., Varley-Campbell, J. et al. (2018). Defining the process to literature searching in systematic reviews: a literature review of guidance and supporting studies. *BMC Med. Res. Methodol.* https://doi.org/10.1186/s12874-018-0545-3.

42. Pradhan, R., Garnick, K., Barkondaj, B. et al. (2018). Inadequate diversity of information resources searched in US-affiliated systematic reviews and meta-analyses: 2005–2016. *J. Clin. Epidemiol.* 102: 50–62.

43. Halfpenny, N.J., Quigley, J.M., Thompson, J.C. et al. (2016). Value and usability of unpublished data sources for systematic reviews and network meta-analyses. *Evid. Based Med.* 21: 208–213.

44. Lefebvre, C., Glanville, J., Briscoe, S. et al. (2019). Chapter 4: searching for and selecting studies. In: *Cochrane Handbook for Systematic*

Reviews of Interventions (eds. J. Higgins, J. Thomas, J. Chandler, et al.). Chichester: Wiley.

45. Biocic, M., Fidahic, M., and Puljak, L. (2019). Reproducibility of search strategies of non-Cochrane systematic reviews published in anaesthesiology journals is suboptimal: primary methodological study. *Br. J. Anaesth.* 122: e79–e81.

46. Mullins, M.M., DeLuca, J.B., Crepaz, N. et al. (2014). Reporting quality of search methods in systematic reviews of HIV behavioral interventions (2000–2010): are the searches clearly explained, systematic and reproducible? *Res. Synth. Methods* 5: 116–130.

47. Koffel, J.B. and Rethlefsen, M.L. (2016). Reproducibility of search strategies is poor in systematic reviews published in high-impact pediatrics, cardiology and surgery journals: a cross-sectional study. *PLoS One* https://doi.org/10.1371/journal.pone.0163309.

48. Franco, J.V.A., Garrote, V.L., Escobar Liquitay, C.M. et al. (2018). Identification of problems in search strategies in Cochrane reviews. *Res. Synth. Methods* 9: 408–416.

49. Salvador-Olivan, J.A., Marco-Cuenca, G., and Arquero-Aviles, R. (2019). Errors in search strategies used in systematic reviews and their effects on information retrieval. *J. Med. Libr. Assoc.* 107: 210–221.

50. Crequit, P., Trinquart, L., Yavchitz, A. et al. (2016). Wasted research when systematic reviews fail to provide a complete and up-to-date evidence synthesis: the example of lung cancer. *BMC Med.* https://doi.org/10.1186/s12916-015-0395-3.

51. Wasiak, J., Tyack, Z., Ware, R. et al. (2017). Poor methodological quality and reporting standards of systematic reviews in burn care management. *Int. Wound J.* 14: 754–763.

52. Pussegoda, K., Turner, L., Garritty, C. et al. (2017). Systematic review adherence to methodological or reporting quality. *Syst. Rev.* https://doi.org/10.1186/s13643-017-0527-2.

53. Liu, P., Qiu, Y., Qian, Y. et al. (2017). Quality of meta-analyses in major leading gastroenterology and hepatology journals: a systematic review. *J. Gastroenterol. Hepatol.* 32: 39–44.

54. Robson, R.C., Pham, B., Hwee, J. et al. (2019). Few studies exist examining methods for selecting studies, abstracting data, and appraising quality in a systematic review. *J. Clin. Epidemiol.* 106: 121–135.

55. Waffenschmidt, S., Knelangen, M., Sieben, W. et al. (2019). Single screening versus conventional double screening for study selection in systematic reviews: a methodological systematic review. *BMC Med. Res. Methodol.* https://doi.org/10.1186/s12874-019-0782-0.

56. Ford, A.C., Guyatt, G.H., Talley, N.J. et al. (2010). Errors in the conduct of systematic reviews of pharmacological interventions for irritable bowel syndrome. *Am. J. Gastroenterol.* 105: 280–288.

57. Mathes, T., Klassen, P., and Pieper, D. (2017). Frequency of data extraction errors and methods to increase data extraction quality: a methodological review. *BMC Med. Res. Methodol.* https://doi.org/10.1186/s12874-017-0431-4.

58. Jones, A.P., Remmington, T., Williamson, P.R. et al. (2005). High prevalence but low impact of data extraction and reporting errors were found in Cochrane systematic reviews. *J. Clin. Epidemiol.* 58: 741–742.

59. Carroll, C., Scope, A., and Kaltenthaler, E. (2013). A case study of binary outcome data extraction across three systematic reviews of hip arthroplasty: errors and differences of selection. *BMC Res. Notes* https://doi.org/10.1186/1756-0500-6-539.

60. Gotzsche, P.C., Hrobjartsson, A., Maric, K. et al. (2007). Data extraction errors in meta-analyses that use standardized mean differences. *JAMA* 298: 430–437.

61. Saldanha, I.J., Lindsley, K., Do, D.V. et al. (2017). Comparison of clinical trial and systematic review outcomes for the 4 most prevalent eye diseases. *JAMA Ophthalmol.* 135: 933–940.

62. Saldanha, I.J., Li, T., Yang, C. et al. (2017). Clinical trials and systematic reviews addressing similar interventions for the same condition do not consider similar outcomes to be important: a case study in HIV/AIDS. *J. Clin. Epidemiol.* 84: 85–94.

63. Mayo-Wilson, E., Fusco, N., Li, T. et al. (2017). Multiple outcomes and analyses in clinical trials create challenges for interpretation and research synthesis. *J. Clin. Epidemiol.* 86: 39–50.

64. Grieve, S., Jones, L., Walsh, N. et al. (2016). What outcome measures are commonly used for complex regional pain syndrome clinical trials? A systematic review of the literature. *Eur. J. Pain* 20: 331–340.

65. Li, T., Mayo-Wilson, E., Fusco, N. et al. (2018). Caveat emptor: the combined effects of multiplicity and selective reporting. *Trials* https://doi.org/10.1186/s13063-018-2888-9.

66. Mayo-Wilson, E., Li, T., Fusco, N. et al. (2017). Cherry-picking by trialists and meta-analysts can drive conclusions about intervention efficacy. *J. Clin. Epidemiol.* 91: 95–110.

67. Whitehead, L., Perkins, G.D., Clarey, A. et al. (2015). A systematic review of the outcomes reported in cardiac arrest clinical trials: the need for a core outcome set. *Resuscitation* 88: 150–157.

68. Yordanov, Y., Dechartres, A., Atal, I. et al. (2018). Avoidable waste of research related to outcome planning and reporting in clinical trials. *BMC Med.* https://doi.org/10.1186/s12916-018-1083-x.

69. Sautenet, B., Contentin, L., Bigot, A. et al. (2016). Strong heterogeneity of outcome reporting in systematic reviews. *J. Clin. Epidemiol.* 75: 93–99.

70. Kicinski, M., Springate, D.A., and Kontopantelis, E. (2015). Publication bias in meta-analyses from the Cochrane database of systematic reviews. *Stat. Med.* 34: 2781–2793.

71. Page, M.J., Forbes, A., Chau, M. et al. (2016). Investigation of bias in meta-analyses due to selective inclusion of trial effect estimates: empirical study. *BMJ Open* https://doi.org/10.1136/bmjopen-2016-011863.

72. Sideri, S., Papageorgiou, S.N., and Eliades, T. (2018). Registration in the international prospective register of systematic reviews (PROSPERO) of systematic review protocols was associated with increased review quality. *J. Clin. Epidemiol.* 100: 103–110.

73. Pandis, N., Fleming, P.S., Worthington, H. et al. (2015). Discrepancies in outcome reporting exist between protocols and published Oral health Cochrane systematic reviews. *PLoS One* https://doi.org/10.1371/journal.pone.0137667.

74. Tricco, A.C., Cogo, E., Page, M.J. et al. (2016). A third of systematic reviews changed or did not specify the primary outcome: a PROSPERO register study. *J. Clin. Epidemiol.* 79: 46–54.

75. Delgado, A.F. and Delgado, A.F. (2017). Inconsistent reporting between meta-analysis protocol and publication – a cross-sectional study. *Anticancer Res.* 37: 5101–5107.

76. Dwan, K., Kirkham, J.J., Williamson, P.R. et al. (2013). Selective reporting of outcomes in randomised controlled trials in systematic reviews of cystic fibrosis. *BMJ Open* https://doi.org/10.1136/bmjopen-2013-002709.

77. Moller, M.H., Ioannidis, J.P.A., and Darmon, M. (2018). Are systematic reviews and meta-analyses still useful research? We are not sure. *Intensive Care Med.* 44: 518–520.

78. Saini, P., Loke, Y.K., Gamble, C. et al. (2014). Selective reporting bias of harm outcomes within studies: findings from a cohort of systematic reviews. *BMJ* https://doi.org/10.1136/bmj.g6501.

79. Parsons, R., Golder, S., and Watt, I. (2019). More than one-third of systematic reviews did not fully report the adverse events outcome. *J. Clin. Epidemiol.* 108: 95–101.

80. Mahady, S.E., Schlub, T., Bero, L. et al. (2015). Side effects are incompletely reported among systematic reviews in gastroenterology. *J. Clin. Epidemiol.* 68: 144–153.

81. Li, L., Xu, C., Deng, K. et al. (2019). The reporting of safety among drug systematic reviews was poor before the implementation of the PRISMA harms checklist. *J. Clin. Epidemiol.* 105: 125–135.

82. Zorzela, L., Loke, Y.K., Ioannidis, J.P. et al. (2016). PRISMA harms checklist: improving harms reporting in systematic reviews. *BMJ* https://doi.org/10.1136/bmj.i157.

83. Detweiler, B.N., Kollmorgen, L.E., Umberham, B.A. et al. (2016). Risk of bias and methodological appraisal practices in systematic reviews published in anaesthetic journals: a meta-epidemiological study. *Anaesthesia* 71: 955–968.

84. Jorgensen, L., Paludan-Muller, A.S., Laursen, D.R. et al. (2016). Evaluation of the Cochrane tool for assessing risk of bias in randomized clinical trials: overview of published comments and analysis of user practice in Cochrane and non-Cochrane reviews. *Syst. Rev.* https://doi.org/10.1186/s13643-016-0259-8.

85. Hopewell, S., Boutron, I., Altman, D.G. et al. (2013). Incorporation of assessments of risk of bias of primary studies in systematic reviews of randomised trials: a cross-sectional study. *BMJ Open* https://doi.org/10.1136/bmjopen-2013-003342.

86. Holihan, J.L., Nguyen, D.H., Flores-Gonzalez, J.R. et al. (2016). A systematic review of randomized controlled trials and reviews in the management of ventral hernias. *J. Surg. Res.* 204: 311–318.

87. Borenstein, M., Hedges, L.V., Higgins, J.P. et al. (2010). A basic introduction to fixed-effect and random-effects models for meta-analysis. *Res. Synth. Methods* 1: 97–111.

88. Rao, G., Lopez-Jimenez, F., Boyd, J. et al. (2017). Methodological standards for meta-analyses and qualitative systematic reviews of cardiac prevention and treatment studies: a scientific statement from the American Heart Association. *Circulation* 136: e172–e194.

89. Riley, R.D., Higgins, J.P., and Deeks, J.J. (2011). Interpretation of random effects meta-analyses. *BMJ* https://doi.org/10.1136/bmj.d549.

90. Bown, M.J. and Sutton, A.J. (2010). Quality control in systematic reviews and meta-analyses. *Eur. J. Vasc. Endovasc. Surg.* 40: 669–677.

91. Page, M.J., Altman, D.G., McKenzie, J.E. et al. (2018). Flaws in the application and interpretation of statistical analyses in systematic reviews of therapeutic interventions were common: a cross-sectional analysis. *J. Clin. Epidemiol.* 95: 7–18.

92. Koletsi, D., Fleming, P.S., Michelaki, I. et al. (2018). Heterogeneity in Cochrane and non-Cochrane meta-analyses in orthodontics. *J. Dent.* 74: 90–94.

93. Riley, R.D., Gates, S., Neilson, J. et al. (2011). Statistical methods can be improved within Cochrane pregnancy and childbirth reviews. *J. Clin. Epidemiol.* 64: 608–618.

94. Baker, W.L., White, C.M., Cappelleri, J.C. et al. (2009). Understanding heterogeneity in meta-analysis: the role of meta-regression. *Int. J. Clin. Pract.* 63: 1426–1434.

95. Gagnier, J.J., Moher, D., Boon, H. et al. (2012). Investigating clinical heterogeneity in systematic reviews: a methodologic review of guidance in the literature. *BMC Med. Res. Methodol.* https://doi.org/10.1186/1471-2288-12-111.

96. Donegan, S., Williams, L., Dias, S. et al. (2015). Exploring treatment by covariate interactions using subgroup analysis and meta-regression in Cochrane reviews: a review of recent practice. *PLoS One* https://doi.org/10.1371/journal.pone.0128804.

97. Chess, L.E. and Gagnier, J.J. (2016). Applicable or non-applicable: investigations of clinical heterogeneity in systematic reviews. *BMC Med. Res. Methodol.* https://doi.org/10.1186/s12874-016-0121-7.

98. Mavridis, D., Chaimani, A., Efthimiou, O. et al. (2014). Addressing missing outcome data in meta-analysis. *Evid. Based Ment. Health* 17: 85–89.

99. Kahale, L.A., Diab, B., Brignardello-Petersen, R. et al. (2018). Systematic reviews do not adequately report or address missing outcome data in their analyses: a methodological survey. *J. Clin. Epidemiol.* 99: 14–23.

100. Akl, E.A., Carrasco-Labra, A., Brignardello-Petersen, R. et al. (2015). Reporting, handling and assessing the risk of bias associated with missing participant data in systematic reviews: a methodological survey. *BMJ Open* https://doi.org/10.1136/bmjopen-2015-009368.

101. Spineli, L.M., Pandis, N., and Salanti, G. (2015). Reporting and handling missing outcome data in mental health: a systematic review of Cochrane systematic reviews and meta-analyses. *Res. Synth. Methods* 6: 175–187.

102. Chalmers, I., Dukan, E., Podolsky, S. et al. (2012). The advent of fair treatment allocation schedules in clinical trials during the 19th and early 20th centuries. *J. R. Soc. Med.* 105: 221–227.

103. IntHout, J., Ioannidis, J.P., Borm, G.F. et al. (2015). Small studies are more heterogeneous than large ones: a meta-meta-analysis. *J. Clin. Epidemiol.* 68: 860–869.

104. von Hippel, P.T. (2015). The heterogeneity statistic I(2) can be biased in small meta-analyses. *BMC Med. Res. Methodol.* https://doi.org/10.1186/s12874-015-0024-z.

105. Turner, R.M., Bird, S.M., and Higgins, J.P. (2013). The impact of study size on meta-analyses: examination of underpowered studies in Cochrane reviews. *PLoS One* https://doi.org/10.1371/journal.pone.0059202.

106. Villas Boas, P.J., Spagnuolo, R.S., Kamegasawa, A. et al. (2013). Systematic reviews showed insufficient evidence for clinical practice in 2004: what about in 2011? The next appeal for the evidence-based medicine age. *J. Eval. Clin. Pract.* 19: 633–637.

107. Goda, Y., Sauer, H., Schondorf, D. et al. (2015). Clinical recommendations of Cochrane reviews in pediatric gastroenterology: systematic analysis. *Pediatr. Int.* 57: 98–106.

108. Willhelm, C., Girisch, W., Gottschling, S. et al. (2013). Systematic Cochrane reviews in neonatology: a critical appraisal. *Pediatr. Neonatol.* 54: 261–266.

109. Ioannidis, J.P. (2016). The mass production of redundant, misleading, and conflicted systematic reviews and meta-analyses. *Milbank Q.* 94: 485–514.

110. Lucenteforte, E., Moja, L., Pecoraro, V. et al. (2015). Discordances originated by multiple meta-analyses on interventions for myocardial infarction: a systematic review. *J. Clin. Epidemiol.* 68: 246–256.

111. Bolland, M.J., Grey, A., and Reid, I.R. (2014). Differences in overlapping meta-analyses of vitamin D supplements and falls. *J. Clin. Endocrinol. Metab.* 99: 4265–4272.

112. Harris, R.G., Neale, E.P., and Ferreira, I. (2019). When poorly conducted systematic reviews and meta-analyses can mislead: a critical appraisal and update of systematic reviews and meta-analyses examining the effects of probiotics in the treatment of functional constipation in children. *Am. J. Clin. Nutr.* 110: 177–195.

113. Prior, M., Hibberd, R., Asemota, N. et al. (2017). Inadvertent P-hacking among trials and systematic reviews of the effect of progestogens in pregnancy? A systematic review and meta-analysis. *Int. J. Obs. Gyn.* 124: 1008–1015.

114. Riva, N., Puljak, L., Moja, L. et al. (2018). Multiple overlapping systematic reviews facilitate the origin of disputes: the case of thrombolytic therapy for pulmonary embolism. *J. Clin. Epidemiol.* 97: 1–13.

115. Page, M.J. and Moher, D. (2016). Mass production of systematic reviews and meta-analyses: an exercise in mega-silliness? *Milbank Q.* 94: 515–519.

116. Doundoulakis, I., Antza, C., Apostolidou-Kiouti, F. et al. (2018). Overview of systematic reviews of non-vitamin K Oral anticoagulants in atrial fibrillation. *Circ. Cardiovasc. Qual. Outcomes* https://doi.org/10.1161/CIRCOUTCOMES.118.004769.

117. Riaz, I.B., Khan, M.S., Riaz, H. et al. (2016). *Am. J. Med.* 129: 339. e11–339.e18.

118. Siontis, K.C., Hernandez-Boussard, T., and Ioannidis, J.P. (2013). Overlapping meta-analyses on the same topic: survey of published studies. *BMJ* https://doi.org/10.1136/bmj.f4501.

119. Niforatos, J.D., Weaver, M., and Johansen, M.E. (2019). Assessment of publication trends of systematic reviews and randomized clinical trials, 1995 to 2017. *JAMA Intern. Med.* 179: 1593–1594.

120. de Vries, Y.A., Roest, A.M., de Jonge, P. et al. (2018). The cumulative effect of reporting and citation biases on the apparent efficacy of treatments: the case of depression. *Psychol. Med.* 48: 2453–2455.

121. Deeks, J.J. (1998). Systematic reviews of published evidence: miracles or minefields? *Ann. Oncol.* 9: 703–709.

CHAPTER 6

Fabrication, Falsification and Spin

The previous chapters have identified that deficiencies frequently occur in the design, conduct and analysis of studies. Many of the defects are associated with biased estimates of treatment benefit and with misleading statistical significance. Lack of knowledge of proper procedures or sloppiness in study conduct is responsible for much wasted research, but it cannot explain why the poor quality studies generally inflate treatment effects and are more likely to produce statistically significant findings. A possible explanation is that wilful manipulation of the research process is common. This chapter explores how often researchers engage in data fabrication, falsification and spin.

FABRICATION

Fabrication involves 'making up data or results and recording or reporting them' [1]. Sometimes this happens on a grand scale. An extreme example is that of Yoshitaka Fujii, a Japanese anaesthetist, who

Evidence in Medicine: The Common Flaws, Why They Occur and How to Prevent Them, First Edition. Iain K Crombie.
© 2021 John Wiley & Sons Ltd. Published 2021 by John Wiley & Sons Ltd.

fabricated all the data in 126 trials and made up much of it for a further 46 studies [2]. The worrying feature of this episode is that, despite clear signs, many years elapsed before the fraud was uncovered. One warning sign was his high frequency of publication, with as many as 20 trials published in a single year [3]. Another was that the data were 'incredibly nice': for example, the frequency of headaches was identical across all groups in 13 trials, and was almost the same in a further 8 studies [4]. Equally surprising patient randomisation resulted in identical numbers in each treatment arm within 17 of the trials. Subsequently, an analysis by Carlisle documented the statistical improbability of the data reported in 168 of Fujii's trials [5]. A detailed investigation by the institutions Fuji was affiliated with, and the Japanese Society of Anaesthetists, finally led to 183 papers being retracted [3].

Several other major league fabricators were identified in the late twentieth and early twenty-first centuries. Joachim Boldt was a German anaesthetist who forged signatures of collaborators, failed to get ethical approval, had incomplete or absent study documentation, and made up the data in 88 papers on the use of hydroxyethyl starch in surgery [6]. Scott Reuben, an American anaesthesiologist, fabricated data in at least 21 trials on drugs for perioperative analgesia [7]. Other researchers have fabricated or falsified data in fields from cancer to cardiovascular disease, and some have been fired or sent to prison for their misconduct [1].

Impact of Fabrication

Data fabrication can distort the scientific evidence, if the proportion of affected trials is large (more specifically the proportion of patients in fraudulent trials compared to the total number of patients in all trials). An example is the use of high-dose mannitol for head injury, in which all of the trials were led by a Brazilian neurosurgeon Julio Cruz [8]. Although a systematic review showed that the high dose appeared more effective than the conventional dose, concerns began to emerge about where and how patients had been recruited to the trials. Subsequent investigation failed to find any evidence that the trials had taken place and the systematic review was withdrawn [8]. The fraudulent trials of the American anaesthesiologist Reuben had less impact. They were included in 25 systematic reviews, but careful analysis showed that findings were only affected when more than 30% of the patients were from the suspect trials [9]. In contrast, Joachim Boldt's studies on fluid resuscitation with hydroxyethyl starch did affect the benefit:harm ratio in systematic reviews: the removal of Boldt's trials showed that resuscitation with hydroxyethyl starch increased the risk of harms, with higher mortality and increased risk of acute kidney disease and sepsis [6].

The consequences of serious research misconduct can be clearly seen in the studies conducted by Yoshihiro Sato. In 2016, concerns were raised about the integrity of the data of 33 trials, and by May 2019, 27 of them had been retracted. A further investigation of the citations of 12 of these studies revealed that they had been mentioned in 1,158 publications, and were included in 68 systematic reviews, other reviews and guidelines [10]. The authors of this investigation judged that 13 of the reviews and guidelines would 'change their findings if the affected trial reports were removed'. Further, the findings from Sato's studies formed part of the justification for eight new trials [10]. Sato's trials 'are likely to have had an adverse impact on clinical care and other research' [10].

Identifying and Managing Data Fabrication

Data fabrication is hard to detect [11]. Most commonly, fraud is reported by whistleblowers, but this relies on other researchers noticing and reporting possible malpractice [12]. An alternative approach is possible. Many of the warning signs were seen in the trials published by Yoshitaka Fujii: such as high rate of publication and a remarkable similarity in the number of patients randomised to the intervention and control groups [13]. These studies also had unexpectedly large, and similar, treatment effects and very low drop-out rates. Based on their experience with the Sato trials, and a review of the literature, one group has compiled a checklist to assist the identification of fraudulent studies [14]. It covers: 'ethical oversight and funding, research productivity and investigator workload, validity of randomization, plausibility of the results and duplicate data reporting' [14]. The tool has been successfully used to identify other problematic studies.

This tool can be used in conjunction with statistical methods that can detect 'anomalies suggestive of fabrication or misconduct' [15, 16]. The idea behind this is that it is hard to fabricate data in ways that are statistically plausible [17]. Statistical methods confirmed the implausibly of the data in the trials of Yoshihiro Sato [13].

Once reported, the investigation of cases of suspected fraud is a major undertaking, taking months if not years, and requiring considerable forensic skills [18]. The costs of the process are not often reported, although in one case this amounted to $525,000 [19] and in another to 'well over a million dollars' [20]. The effort involved, and the potential damage to their reputations, may deter universities from undertaking full investigations of potential misconduct [20]. One recent study found 'important deficiencies in the quality and reporting of institutional investigation of concerns about the integrity of a large body of research' [21].

Reluctance to Report

One reason that fraud may flourish is that people are reluctant to report it. Several studies have shown that awareness of research misconduct does not often lead to it being reported [22, 23]. Researchers are willing to admit to their reluctance to report fraud. Among Dutch biomedical scientists 21% admitted that they had ignored research misconduct by colleagues [24]. A survey of research coordinators in the US revealed that 48% would not report it, and a further 27% would ask the Principal Investigator to do so [22].

One reason for doing nothing is that whistleblowing is a fraught activity; those reporting misconduct frequently feel stigmatised and can suffer adverse effects on physical and mental health [23, 25]. One whistleblower described the experiences of a group of graduate students who raised concerns [26]. Following 'months of tortured deliberation' they reported the misconduct of their supervisor. The subsequent investigation took several months, at the end of which the supervisor resigned and the research laboratory was closed. The graduate students were advised to find a new research home, leading some students to abandon their PhDs [26].

A paper entitled 'No one likes a snitch' sheds light on more unpleasant potential consequences: concerns about retribution [27]. The 'realistic fear of retaliation' is a deterrent to the potential whistle-blower [28]. A more recent study expanded on this, showing that: reporting was thought to be much easier if the colleague were junior to the whistleblower; previous negative experience was a deterrent; and providing evidence for the claim could be difficult [29]. Upholding the integrity of science can come at a high price, with those reporting misconduct being given little protection [23, 25].

FALSIFICATION

Falsification is the wilful distortion of some data or results [30], usually with the intent to deceive or mislead. Even distinguished scientists may have been guilty of this. A reanalysis of Gregor Mendel's famous studies on the laws of inheritance concluded that 'the data of most, if not all, of the experiments have been falsified so as to agree closely with Mendel's expectations' [31].

The number of researchers who falsify or manipulate some of their data is not large, but could still be a cause for concern. A systematic review published in 2009 found that about 2% of researchers had fabricated, falsified or modified data and 14% had observed such practices by colleagues [30]. Subsequent surveys have reported similar results with estimates 0.6%, 1.4 % and 2.4% for personally falsifying data [32–34] and 4% and 27% for that behaviour in colleagues [35, 36].

QUESTIONABLE RESEARCH PRACTICES

Questionable research practices, such as excluding selected data points or rounding down p-values, are common. These misbehaviours are not included within the definition of falsification [30] and are commonly reported separately in surveys. A 2009 systematic review reported that up to 34% of researchers had engaged in them and up to 72% had observed other researchers doing so [30]. Table 6.1 shows the reported frequencies of potentially serious questionable research practices.

TABLE 6.1   Frequency of questionable research practices.

Action	Frequency	References
Dropping data points based on gut feeling	15.3%, 15%	Martinson [37], Godecharle [35]
Deleting data points after the analysis	13%, 38%, 42%	Artino [34], John [32], Janke [38]
Selectively reporting findings	12%, 24%, 63%	Artino [34], Boulbes [36], John [32]
Reporting an unexpected finding as a predicted hypothesis	20%, 20%, 27%, 41%	Artino [34], Tijink [24], John [32], Janke [38]
Rounding down a p-value	3%, 8%, 22%	Artino [34], Janke [38], John [32]
Collecting more data after seeing the results were almost significant	14%, 22.6%, 56%	Artino [34], Janke [38], John [32]

A nationwide survey of doctoral students sheds additional light on these findings. It found that 13% of respondents agreed it was acceptable to omit contradictory findings if this expedited publication [39]. In addition 10% would falsify or fabricate data if they were confident of their findings, and it would lead to publication. Misbehaviour may become acceptable to some researchers when it could promote their careers [40].

SPIN

Spin in research papers has been defined as 'reporting that could distort the interpretation of results and mislead readers' [41]. One aim of spin is to put 'negative findings in a more palatable way to editors, journals, patients, funders and readers' [42]. It is seen in reports that make claims of 'yet another revolutionary clinical innovation' [43]. Spin can also be used for the 'beautification of methods' [44]. Spin is common in clinical trials, with one review concluding that a median of 57% of published trials contained instances of it [45]. Spin can have seriously adverse effects: as one journal editor remarked: 'spin kills science' [42]. Many techniques are used to spin.

Focussing on Misleading Significance

A common technique is to highlight a significant secondary outcome when the primary outcome was not significant. Several studies have explored the frequency of this type of spin among trials with a non-significant primary outcome. Spin occurred in 40% of trials in obstetrics and gynaecology [46], in 28% of analgesic trials [47], 11% of wound care trials [48] and 5% of general medical trials [41]. Other spin techniques were to emphasise changes over time rather than the comparison between groups, to focus on subgroup analyses, or to emphasise significant finding from an interim analysis instead of the non-significant final analysis [41, 47, 49, 50].

Drawing Misleading Conclusions

Drawing conclusions that do not reflect the study findings is a major problem [51]. Many trials make exaggerated claims. Among trials in wound care research, 30% claimed the treatment was effective when the primary outcome was non-significant [48]. Similarly, in oncology trials, biased reporting was often used 'to imply benefit of the experimental treatment' [52]. In a study of surgical trials, although most articles acknowledged the non-significant primary outcome, 23% recommended the use of the intervention [53].

Another approach is to claim that a treatment was equally effective as the standard treatment, when the analysis simply failed to show a significant difference. This is the classic confusion of lack of evidence for a difference with evidence that there is no difference [54]. This type of confusion is common: it was seen in 76% of abstracts of trials evaluating robotic colorectal surgery [55] and in 43% of laparoscopic lower gastrointestinal surgery trials [56]. It occurred, but less commonly, in trials of wound care (21%) [48], analgesics (13%) [47] and general medical trials (14%) [41].

Misleading Abstracts

The abstract is important. The results and conclusions it contains are accessible online, even if the rest of the paper is not. The abstract, with the title, is used by journal editors to decide if a submitted manuscript should be sent out for peer review [57]. This may be why spin is particularly common in abstracts. For example, 8 out of 10 systematic reviews on chronic pain had abstracts with some form of spin [58] as did many abstracts of trials in psychiatry and psychology (56%) [59], obesity 47% [49] and surgery (40%) [53]. An earlier review of such studies found that between 5% and 45% of papers had major inconsistencies between the abstracts and the full reports [60].

Words to Mislead

The words used to describe results may influence their interpretation. Recent years have seen a marked increase in the use of positive terms such as novel, excellent, prominent, remarkable and unprecedented in the titles and abstracts of papers [61, 62]. One study evaluating the use of adjectives in abstracts identified a frequent use of imprecise terms such as meaningful, favourable, promising and useful [63]. As well as individual words, phrases may be used to increase the apparent importance of findings: 'provides strong evidence', 'we believe our study makes it clear', or 'shows that [the treatment] is very effective' [64]. Another approach is to describe a non-significant result as showing 'a trend to significance' [49]. A website has collated over 400 such phrases from peer-reviewed journals: some intriguing ones were 'as good as significant', 'partly significant', 'probably significant' and 'significantly significant' [65]. None were statistically significant.

Misleading terms are often used when evaluating harms. The phrase 'safe and well tolerated', which was used in over 5,000 trials published between 1990 and 2015, has been strongly criticised [66]. It an unjustified generalisation, as the sample size of most clinical trials is much too small to allow any assessment of safety. A review of 122 trials of cancer drugs found that 43% used terms that downplayed harms [67]. Commonly used terms were 'acceptable', 'manageable' and 'favourable toxicity profile'. The problem is that the researchers are assigning these labels to harms, rather than asking for the patient's assessment of them.

RETRACTIONS

When serious errors or misconduct have been identified in a published study, a notice of retraction can be published by the relevant journal. Only a small proportion of published papers is retracted, about 0.02% of all articles [68], although its frequency is increasing [69, 70]. The reasons for retraction vary across studies, with fraud or misconduct, unintentional error and duplicate publication being common [69–72]. Not all instances of serious misconduct result in a retraction: among cases of misconduct confirmed by the US Office of Research Integrity, 20% did not lead to a notice of retraction [73].

On average papers are retracted about two years after they were published [72, 74]. Retracted papers continue to be cited after a notice of retraction has been published, suggesting that the claims of the disgraced study are still taken at face value [74–76]. The process for reporting retraction is not well publicised, and journal editors are sometimes reluctant or slow to take action [77–79].

DISCUSSION

The fabrication of large amounts of data is thought to be rare, and often comes to light because observant individuals become suspicious. It is likely that many cases are not detected because researchers are unwilling to report such serious misbehaviours. Statistical methods can help detect large-scale fabrication of data, and if these tools were widely used many more cases of fraud might be detected.

Surveys show that the self-reported frequency of data fabrication is low. These studies suffer from the handicap that researchers may be reluctant to admit to behaviours that are widely considered unacceptable [1, 30]. Thus the true frequencies of fabrication may be higher than reported.

Questionable research practices have been described as 'strategies that aim to increase the chance to publish at the cost of scientific accuracy' [38]. The proportion of researchers who engage in these practices ranges from a few per cent to over 60%, depending on the type of behaviour involved. The high frequencies of questionable research practices suggests considerable potential to distort study findings; as Fanelli commented 'their negative impact on research can be dramatic' [30]. The cumulative effects of falsifying some data and manipulating the statistical analysis to produce a desired result could lead to substantial bias. The ubiquity of questionable behaviours suggests that the findings of many published research studies will be affected.

Individuals often believe that other researchers are more likely to engage in questionable research practices than they are. A systematic review found that the frequency of observing others engaging in questionable research practices (72%) was more than double that of the self-reports (34%) [30]. This view that most people are doing it could be creating an environment in which 'some questionable research practices may constitute the prevailing research norm' [32].

Spin is common in research articles, and can influence judgements about the effectiveness of treatments [80]. It produces 'an abundance of scientific articles with catchy titles, often exaggerated abstracts and little scientific substance' [81]. One explanation for spin is unconscious prejudice, possibly resulting from a desire to have an effective treatment [82]. Other less innocent motives are that authors spin their findings to increase the chance of being published or to be more widely cited [44, 61]. Spin has been placed at one end of a hype-hypocrisy-falsification-fakery continuum, with the suggestion that 'It is but another step down from the grey hinterland of hype into the dark underworld of deliberate falsification' [83].

This chapter has shown that researchers frequently engage in activities to make undistinguished results appear novel and important. The key question emerging from these findings is why the prevalence of these misbehaviours is so high. The next chapter explores possible explanations for these behaviours.

REFERENCES

1. George, S.L. (2016). Research misconduct and data fraud in clinical trials: prevalence and causal factors. *Int. J. Clin. Oncol.* 21: 15–21.

2. George, S.L. and Buyse, M. (2015). Data fraud in clinical trials. *Clin. Investig.* 5: 161–173.

3. Tramer, M.R. (2013). The Fujii story: a chronicle of naive disbelief. *Eur. J. Anaesthesiol.* 30: 195–198.

4. Kranke, P., Apfel, C.C., Roewer, N. et al. (2000). Reported data on granisetron and postoperative nausea and vomiting by Fujii et al. are incredibly nice! *Anesth. Analg.* 90: 1004–1007.

5. Carlisle, J.B. (2012). The analysis of 168 randomised controlled trials to test data integrity. *Anaesthesia* 67: 521–537.

6. Wise, J. (2013). Boldt: the great pretender. *BMJ* https://doi .org/10.1136/bmj.f1738.

7. Shafer, S.L. (2009). Tattered threads. *Anesth. Analg.* 108: 1361–1363.

8. Roberts, I., Smith, R., and Evans, S. (2007). Doubts over head injury studies. *BMJ* 334: 392–394.

9. Marret, E., Elia, N., Dahl, J.B. et al. (2009). Susceptibility to fraud in systematic reviews: lessons from the Reuben case. *Anesthesiology* 111: 1279–1289.

10. Avenell, A., Stewart, F., Grey, A. et al. (2019). An investigation into the impact and implications of published papers from retracted research: systematic search of affected literature. *BMJ Open* https:// doi.org/10.1136/bmjopen-2019-031909.

11. Tavare, A. (2011). Managing research misconduct: is anyone getting it right? *BMJ* https://doi.org/10.1136/bmj.d8212.

12. Breen, K.J. (2016). Research misconduct: time for a re-think? *Intern. Med. J.* 46: 728–733.

13. Bolland, M.J., Avenell, A., Gamble, G.D. et al. (2016). Systematic review and statistical analysis of the integrity of 33 randomized controlled trials. *Neurology* 87: 2391–2402.

14. Grey, A., Bolland, M.J., Avenell, A. et al. (2020). Check for publication integrity before misconduct. *Nature* 577: 167–169.

15. Knepper, D., Lindblad, A.S., Sharma, G. et al. (2016). Statistical monitoring in clinical trials: best practices for detecting data anomalies suggestive of fabrication or misconduct. *Ther. Innov. Regul. Sci.* 50: 144–154.
16. Herson, J. (2016). Strategies for dealing with fraud in clinical trials. *Int. J. Clin. Oncol.* 21: 22–27.
17. Sakamoto, J. and Buyse, M. (2016). Fraud in clinical trials: complex problem, simple solutions? *Int. J. Clin. Oncol.* 21: 13–14.
18. Chalmers, I. and Haines, A. (2011). Commentary: skilled forensic capacity needed to investigate allegations of research misconduct. *BMJ* https://doi.org/10.1136/bmj.d3977.
19. Michalek, A.M., Hutson, A.D., Wicher, C.P. et al. (2010). The costs and underappreciated consequences of research misconduct: a case study. *PLoS Med.* https://doi.org/10.1371/journal.pmed.1000318.
20. Wager, E. (2012). Who is responsible for investigating suspected research misconduct? *Anaesthesia* 67: 462–466.
21. Grey, A., Bolland, M., Gamble, G. et al. (2019). Quality of reports of investigations of research integrity by academic institutions. *Res. Integr. Peer Rev.* https://doi.org/10.1186/s41073-019-0062-x.
22. Pryor, E.R., Habermann, B., and Broome, M.E. (2007). Scientific misconduct from the perspective of research coordinators: a national survey. *J. Med. Ethics* 33: 365–369.
23. Resnik, D.B. and Shamoo, A.E. (2017). Fostering research integrity. *Account Res.* 24: 367–372.
24. Tijdink, J.K., Bouter, L.M., Veldkamp, C.L. et al. (2016). Personality traits are associated with research misbehavior in Dutch scientists: a cross-sectional study. *PLoS One* https://doi.org/10.1371/journal.pone.0163251.
25. Bouter, L.M. and Hendrix, S. (2017). Both whistleblowers and the scientists they accuse are vulnerable and deserve protection. *Account Res.* 24: 359–366.
26. Allen, M. and Dowell, R. (2013). Retrospective reflections of a whistleblower: opinions on misconduct responses. *Account Res.* 20: 339–348.
27. Redman, B. and Caplan, A. (2015). No one likes a snitch. *Sci. Eng. Ethics* 21: 813–819.

28. Kornfeld, D.S. (2012). Perspective: research misconduct: the search for a remedy. *Acad. Med.* 87: 877–882.

29. Satalkar, P. and Shaw, D. (2018). Is failure to raise concerns about misconduct a breach of integrity? Researchers' reflections on reporting misconduct. *Account. Res.* 25: 311–339.

30. Fanelli, D. (2009). How many scientists fabricate and falsify research? A systematic review and meta-analysis of survey data. *PLoS One* https://doi.org/10.1371/journal.pone.0005738.

31. Fisher, R. (1936). Has Mendel's work been rediscovered? *Ann. Sci.* 1: 115–137.

32. John, L.K., Loewenstein, G., and Prelec, D. (2012). Measuring the prevalence of questionable research practices with incentives for truth telling. *Psychol. Sci.* 23: 524–532.

33. Hofmann, B. and Holn, S. (2019). Research integrity: environment, experience, or ethos? *Res. Ethics* 15: 1–13.

34. Artino, A.R. Jr., Driessen, E.W., and Maggio, L.A. (2019). Ethical shades of gray: international frequency of scientific misconduct and questionable research practices in health professions education. *Acad. Med.* 94: 76–84.

35. Godecharle, S., Fieuws, S., Nemery, B. et al. (2018). Scientists still behaving badly? A survey within industry and universities. *Sci. Eng. Ethics* 24: 1697–1717.

36. Boulbes, D.R., Costello, T., Baggerly, K. et al. (2018). A survey on data reproducibility and the effect of publication process on the ethical reporting of laboratory research. *Clin. Cancer Res.* 24: 3447–3455.

37. Martinson, B.C., Anderson, M.S., and de Vries, R. (2005). Scientists behaving badly. *Nature* 435: 737–738.

38. Janke, S., Daumiller, M., and Rudert, S.C. (2019). Dark pathways to achievement in science: researchers' achievement goals predict engagement in questionable research practices. *Soc. Psychol. Personal. Sci.* 10: 783–791.

39. Hofmann, B., Helgesson, G., Juth, N. et al. (2015). Scientific dishonesty: a survey of doctoral students at the major medical faculties in Sweden and Norway. *J. Empir. Res. Hum. Res. Ethics* 10: 380–388.

40. Bruton, S.V., Medlin, M., Brown, M. et al. (2020). Personal motivations and systemic incentives: scientists on questionable research practices. *Sci. Eng. Ethics* 26: 1531–1547.

41. Boutron, I., Dutton, S., Ravaud, P. et al. (2010). Reporting and interpretation of randomized controlled trials with statistically nonsignificant results for primary outcomes. *JAMA* 303: 2058–2064.

42. Harvey, L.A. (2015). Spin kills science. *Spinal Cord* 53: 417.

43. Evers, J.L.H. (2018). Take a break! *Hum. Reprod.* 33: 769.

44. Boutron, I. and Ravaud, P. (2018). Misrepresentation and distortion of research in biomedical literature. *Proc. Natl. Acad. Sci. U. S. A.* 115: 2613–2619.

45. Chiu, K., Grundy, Q., and Bero, L. (2017). 'Spin' in published biomedical literature: a methodological systematic review. *PLoS Biol.* https://doi.org/10.1371/journal.pbio.2002173.

46. Turrentine, M. (2017). It's all how you 'spin' it: interpretive bias in research findings in the obstetrics and gynecology literature. *Obstet. Gynecol.* 129: 239–242.

47. Gewandter, J.S., McKeown, A., McDermott, M.P. et al. (2015). Data interpretation in analgesic clinical trials with statistically nonsignificant primary analyses: an ACTTION systematic review. *J. Pain* 16: 3–10.

48. Lockyer, S., Hodgson, R., Dumville, J.C. et al. (2013). *Trials* https://doi.org/10.1186/1745-6215-14-371.

49. Austin, J., Smith, C., Natarajan, K. et al. (2018). *Clin. Obes.* 9: e12292.

50. Motosko, C.C., Ault, A.K., Kimberly, L.L. et al. (2019). Analysis of spin in the reporting of studies of topical treatments of photoaged skin. *J. Am. Acad. Dermatol.* 80: 516–522.

51. Gerrits, R.G., Jansen, T., Mulyanto, J. et al. (2019). Occurrence and nature of questionable research practices in the reporting of messages and conclusions in international scientific health services research publications: a structured assessment of publications authored by researchers in the Netherlands. *BMJ Open* https://doi.org/10.1136/bmjopen-2018-027903.

52. Vera-Badillo, F.E., Napoleone, M., Krzyzanowska, M.K. et al. (2016). Bias in reporting of randomised clinical trials in oncology. *Eur. J. Cancer* 61: 29–35.

53. Arunachalam, L., Hunter, I.A., and Killeen, S. (2017). Reporting of randomized controlled trials with statistically nonsignificant primary outcomes published in high-impact surgical journals. *Ann. Surg.* 265: 1141–1145.

54. Altman, D.G. and Bland, J.M. (1995). Absence of evidence is not evidence of absence. *BMJ* https://doi.org/10.1136/bmj.311.7003.485.

55. Patel, S.V., Van Koughnett, J.A., Howe, B. et al. (2015). Spin is common in studies assessing robotic colorectal surgery: an assessment of reporting and interpretation of study results. *Dis. Colon Rectum* 58: 878–884.

56. Patel, S.V., Chadi, S.A., Choi, J. et al. (2013). The use of 'spin' in laparoscopic lower GI surgical trials with nonsignificant results: an assessment of reporting and interpretation of the primary outcomes. *Dis. Colon Rectum* 56: 1388–1394.

57. Cals, J.W., Kotz, D. et al. (2013). *J. Clin. Epidemiol.* 66: 585.

58. Nascimento, D.P., Gonzalez, G.Z., Araujo, A.C. et al. (2019). Eight out of every ten abstracts of low Back pain systematic reviews presented spin and inconsistencies with the full text: an analysis of 66 systematic reviews. *J. Orthop. Sports Phys. Ther.* 50: 17–23.

59. Jellison, S., Roberts, W., Bowers, A. et al. (2019). Evaluation of spin in abstracts of papers in psychiatry and psychology journals. *BMJ Evid. Based Med.* 25: 178–181.

60. Li, G., Abbade, L.P.F., Nwosu, I. et al. (2017). A scoping review of comparisons between abstracts and full reports in primary biomedical research. *BMC Med. Res. Methodol.* https://doi.org/10.1186/s12874-017-0459-5.

61. Vinkers, C.H., Tijdink, J.K., and Otte, W.M. (2015). Use of positive and negative words in scientific PubMed abstracts between 1974 and 2014: retrospective analysis. *BMJ* https://doi.org/10.1136/bmj.h6467.

62. Lerchenmueller, M.J., Sorenson, O., and Jena, A.B. (2019). Gender differences in how scientists present the importance of their research: observational study. *BMJ* https://doi.org/10.1136/bmj.l6573.

63. Cepeda, M.S., Berlin, J.A., Glasser, S.C. et al. (2015). Use of adjectives in abstracts when reporting results of randomized, controlled trials from industry and academia. *Drugs R D.* 15: 85–139.

64. Cummings, P. and Rivara, F.P. (2012). Spin and boasting in research articles. *Arch. Pediatr. Adolesc. Med.* 166: 1099–1100.
65. Anonymous: Probable Error. https://mchankins.wordpress.com/2013/04/21/still-not-significant-2` (accessed 17 May 2020).
66. Lineberry, N., Berlin, J.A., Mansi, B. et al. (2016). *BMJ* https://doi.org/10.1136/bmj.i5078.
67. Gyawali, B., Shimokata, T., Honda, K. et al. (2018). Reporting harms more transparently in trials of cancer drugs. *BMJ* https://doi.org/10.1136/bmj.k4383.
68. Hesselmann, F., Graf, V., Schmidt, M. et al. (2017). The visibility of scientific misconduct: a review of the literature on retracted journal articles. *Curr. Sociol.* 65: 814–845.
69. Bozzo, A., Bali, K., Evaniew, N. et al. (2017). Retractions in cancer research: a systematic survey. *Res. Integr. Peer Rev.* https://doi.org/10.1186/s41073-017-0031-1.
70. Wang, T., Xing, Q.R., Wang, H. et al. (2019). Retracted publications in the biomedical literature from open Access Journals. *Sci. Eng. Ethics* 25: 855–868.
71. Li, G., Kamel, M., Jin, Y. et al. (2018). Exploring the characteristics, global distribution and reasons for retraction of published articles involving human research participants: a literature survey. *J. Multidiscip. Healthc.* 11: 39–47.
72. Wang, J., Ku, J.C., Alotaibi, N.M. et al. (2017). Retraction of neurosurgical publications: a systematic review. *World Neurosurg.* 103: 809–814.e1.
73. Drimer-Batca, D. and Iaccarino, J. (2019). Status of retraction notices for biomedical publications associated with research misconduct. *Res. Ethics* 15: 1–5.
74. Bar-Ilan, J. and Halevi, G. (2017). Post retraction citations in context: a case study. *Scientometrics* 113: 547–565.
75. Lu, S.F., Jin, G.Z., Uzzi, B. et al. (2013). *Sci. Report.* 3: 3146.
76. Mott, A., Fairhurst, C., and Torgerson, D. (2019). Assessing the impact of retraction on the citation of randomized controlled trial reports: an interrupted time-series analysis. *J. Health Serv. Res. Policy* 24: 44–51.

77. Allison, D.B., Brown, A.W., George, B.J. et al. (2016). Reproducibility: a tragedy of errors. *Nature* 530: 27–29.

78. Kupferschmidt, K. (2018). Tide of lies. *Science* 361: 636–641.

79. Wiedermann, C.J. (2018). Inaction over retractions of identified fraudulent publications: ongoing weakness in the system of scientific self-correction. *Account Res.* 25: 239–253.

80. Boutron, I., Altman, D.G., Hopewell, S. et al. (2014). Impact of spin in the abstracts of articles reporting results of randomized controlled trials in the field of cancer: the SPIIN randomized controlled trial. *J. Clin. Oncol.* 32: 4120–4126.

81. Madsen, R.R. (2019). Scientific impact and the quest for visibility. *FEBS J.* 286: 3968–3974.

82. Mahtani, K.R. (2016). 'Spin' in reports of clinical research. *Evid. Based Med.* 21: 201–202.

83. Hopf, H., Matlin, S.A., Mehta, G. et al. (2020). Blocking the hype-hypocrisy-falsification-fakery pathway is needed to safeguard science. *Angew. Chem. Int. Ed.* 59: 2150–2154.

CHAPTER 7

Why Do Researchers Falsify Data or Manipulate Study Findings?

This chapter explores the causes of data falsification and questionable research practices, to identify why they occur. It assesses whether the research environment may contribute to misconduct and whether the system of research oversight is sufficiently robust to detect misconduct. The chapter also explores the role of individual level factors in questionable research practices.

THE RESEARCH ENVIRONMENT

Science is a highly competitive field in which large numbers of researchers compete for limited research funding and for a limited number of jobs [1–3]. Researchers think that competition for funding and lack of jobs are the main challenges to career progression

Evidence in Medicine: The Common Flaws, Why They Occur and How to Prevent Them, First Edition. Iain K Crombie.
© 2021 John Wiley & Sons Ltd. Published 2021 by John Wiley & Sons Ltd.

[4]. A common view is that researchers need to 'bullshit or bluff or lie or embellish in order to get grants' [5].

Appointments, promotion and tenure of researchers are based mainly on published papers [6, 7]. This places researchers under a strong pressure to publish [8], particularly in prestigious journals [2, 9]. The pressure to publish is a major cause of stress, particularly among early and middle career researchers; it also leads to 'a disproportionate focus on positive and spectacular results' [10].

In recent years, striving for excellence has become the dominant theme of the research environment [11]. Excellence is essentially comparative: an individual is judged excellent when their research outputs are better than most others. This contributes to a climate of hypercompetition, in which scientific integrity suffers [3]. Competition has always been a feature of science, because it was thought to encourage researchers to excel and to disseminate their findings quickly [12]. But excessive competition 'compromises the integrity of the research enterprise', by encouraging game-playing, interference with peer review and questionable research conduct [13]. It may also stifle creativity [12]. In an environment of hypercompetition, researchers feel that they must 'emphasise, overstate, embellish or fabricate to appear more excellent than their competitors' [11]. They believe that 'researchers' careers depend more on publishing results with "impact" than on publishing results that are correct' [14].

A common view is that to publish in a leading journal, studies have to produce 'clean stories and immaculate data' [9], to have findings that are novel and statistically significant [15, 16], and that 'represent a major, and possibly newsworthy, advance in knowledge' [2]. There is some truth behind this: interviews with editors revealed that one wanted 'papers to make your journal look good' and another said 'we don't publish negative trials' [17]. It has been suggested that journals welcome eye-catching papers because these will be highly cited and thus boost the journal's impact factor [18]. Some leading journals are explicit about this: the guidance to potential authors includes phrases such as 'papers should present novel and broadly important data, syntheses or concepts' and 'the results seem novel, arresting (illuminating, unexpected or surprising)' [19]. The guidelines of the International Committee of Medical Journal Editors advise authors to 'emphasize the new and important aspects of your study' [20].

Impact Factors

The impact factor of the journal in which a paper has been published is a widely used measure of the quality and value of a research study. The emphasis given to impact factor leads to what has been termed impact factor mania, in which researchers show an excessive enthusiasm for publishing in prestigious journals [9]. Getting papers into top-rated journals has been likened to joining the golden club, bringing 'job opportunities, invitations to speak, grants, promotions and even cash bonuses and prizes' [21].

The impact factor has been widely criticised because it does not measure the quality or importance of individual studies, but instead is an average of how often all the papers published in the journal are cited by other papers [3, 22, 23]. It evaluates a study by 'the journal where the work is published rather than the content of the work itself' [9]. As Zhang and colleagues put it, 'science deserves to be judged by its contents, not by its wrapping' [24].

Another weakness of impact factors is that journals, which are mainly for-profit businesses, can manipulate their impact factors [25]. Several techniques can be employed such as encouraging authors to cite papers in their journal, setting up cross-journal citation cartels, accepting papers on hot topics and rejecting those with negative findings, publishing systematic reviews because they are often highly cited, and attracting articles from prestigious scientists or from large research groups [25–27]. Although widely used, the impact factor is at best a blunt instrument for assessing research activity.

Perverse Incentives

The high premium on novel significant results creates a pressure to massage results [8, 9] or to convert an accidental finding into a predicted hypothesis [15]. This process of significance chasing leads to many false positive studies being published [16]. As Grimes and colleagues concluded the 'fixation in top tier journals on significant or positive findings tends to drive trustworthiness of published science down, and is more likely to select for false positives and fraudulent results' [28].

The competitive nature of the research environment, and a reward system based on publication in high impact journals, exacerbates the problems of poor quality and dubious research. The publish or perish climate encourages 'hasty, low quality, incomplete research with the aim of maximising the number of papers from a single study' [29]. Often statistical analysis is motivated more by the desire to get a paper published than to report what was really found [30].

Not all researchers try to massage their studies to produce spectacular findings. When the results are not what were hoped for, many conclude that they will not 'waste their time trying to publish a manuscript that they know will be rejected' [31]. A survey of researchers with unpublished trials found that many were less likely to write up a paper when the results were not interesting, not statistically significant or negative [32]. An overview of such studies found that together unimportant or negative results, fear of rejection and lack of time or low priority accounted for just over one half of the unpublished studies [33].

A different kind of perverse incentive is the system of rewards to individuals. In some countries substantial cash sums are given to individuals for publishing in prestigious journals [34, 35]. Successful academics, those with frequently cited papers in high impact journals, can be given special funding to support their research [36]. The motivation is to boost the scientific ranking of the host institution, but there is an unintended consequence. It can give rise to the Matthew effect ('For whoever has, to him more shall be given' Matthew chapter 25 verse 29) in which successful researchers are given greater support for their research [37]. It will reward the truly excellent, but will also support the less scrupulous to continue manipulating their research. The current incentive system creates the conditions for scientific misconduct to flourish.

Gaming the System

The use of publication metrics to evaluate research output encourages gaming, the manipulation and enhancement of these metrics to gain a high rating [38]. The process of rating individuals is potentially counterproductive: 'when we believe that will be judged by silly criteria we will adapt and behave in silly ways' [39]. This gives rise to the performance paradox, in which individuals target their efforts to improve their scores on the assessment measures, rather than on conducting high quality research [40]. It provides another demonstration of Goodhart's Law, that 'when a measure becomes a target it ceases to be a good measure' [41].

Researchers have been very creative in their efforts to game citation metrics. One study listed 33 strategies to increase the rate at which papers are cited, such as: set up a blog, join an academic social network, add recent papers to your e-mail signature and deposit your paper in an open access repository [42]. Such efforts have been described as 'marketing campaigns where researchers advertise themselves' [43]. Other, less reputable, techniques are described below.

Self-citation is a simple method of increasing a paper's citations, in which each new paper cites several of the author's previous publications [44]. For example, when a citation threshold was set for the promotion of Italian researchers, they responded by substantially increasing the number self-citations [45]. An extension of this is citation rings, in which a group of individuals agree to cite each other's papers [46, 47]. A variation on self-citation is coercive citation, in which peer reviewers request that the author of a submitted paper includes one or more of their published papers [44, 48]. One reviewer, whose own work was highly cited, took coercive citation to the extreme, by requiring that authors reference dozens of his papers [49]. Journal editors can also engage in coercive citation by requesting citations of papers published in their journal [50].

Salami slicing is the technique in which, rather than being presented in a single paper, the results are packaged into two or more publications. Researchers chop up the data so that each paper contains the 'minimum publishable unit of research', thereby boosting their total publications [51]. Clinical trials frequently produce multiple papers with the primary results paper being followed by several others [52]. These often test different hypotheses to that of the main paper, and almost always report statistically significant findings, raising concerns about multiple testing and the increased risk of spuriously significant findings [52]. A variant on salami slicing is duplicate publication, in which there is major overlap in the results of two papers [51]. The redundancy of the second paper can be concealed by changing the title and making small alterations to the data presented.

The pressure to publish may encourage a focus on hot topics, so that the importance of the subject, rather than the scientific value of the study, ensures publication in a leading journal [53]. This was seen clearly during the Covid 19 pandemic, where 'a deluge of poor quality research' was 'sabotaging an effective evidence based response' [54]. Over 1,000 trials of treatments of Covid 19 were registered on http://ClinicalTrials.gov within five months of the start of the outbreak. There was considerable redundancy across these studies; for example 145 trials evaluated the effect of the drug hydroxychloroquine [54]. Many of these studies were small and based on limited registration data and, there was evidence of outcome switching. The findings were often published as preprints and many were poorly reported. A similar redundancy has occurred with systematic reviews. For example five systematic reviews of the effect of face masks were conducted in parallel [54].

Deliberately conducting small studies with poor methods is another way to enhance a publication record [30, 55]. Conducting several small studies will result in many more papers than would one large rigorous study. Just by chance some of these small studies will produce unexpected and spuriously significant findings, and may be more likely to be published in journals seeking novel findings. Researchers who adopt this strategy will quickly gain impressive publication lists, which will lead to promotion, to more research grants and to more poor quality studies. This process has been termed 'the natural selection of bad science' [30]. It succeeds because of the emphasis on exciting new findings, rather than rigorous methods.

RESEARCH OVERSIGHT

The research system is based on trust, with the assumption that researchers are honest, impartial and objective [56–58]. As Relman commented '[Science] is intensely skeptical about the possibility of error, but totally trusting about the possibility of fraud' [59]. Trust leads to a presumption that data have not been fabricated, that high quality methods have been used, that the analysis has not been manipulated and that the conclusions are based on the findings. The high frequency of data falsification and questionable research practices suggests that the research environment is sufficiently permissive to allow motivated individuals to cheat: 'misconduct may be easier for scientists because the system operates on trust' [60]. Despite several initiatives to improve research integrity, much remains to be done before trust in research can be assumed [61–64]. In the current system, 'the biggest mistake of all, then, is taking evidence on trust and without checking it' [65].

Peer Review

Almost all medical journals have a system of peer review, which is intended to 'ensure the quality and correctness of the scientific literature' [66]. In this process, independent experts comment on the suitability of submitted manuscripts for publication [67]. Although a well-established practice, there is a long-standing, vigorous and polarised debate about the value of peer review [68]. Some see peer review as a 'gold standard for scientific scholarship' [69] while others assert it is 'of questionable value' [70]. This diversity of view is understandable, given the paucity of evidence for the effectiveness of peer review [71].

Peer review has a number of weaknesses. The system relies on trust: 'it is not the role of journals to police research integrity or determine if misconduct has occurred' [68]. In fairness, it is particularly difficult for reviewers to detect fabricated data [66]. Another problem is that most journals do not specifically request comments on risk of bias from their reviewers [67]. There are also concerns that the peer reviewers are not adequately trained to detect deficiencies in research studies [72, 73]. It is thought that peer review often focuses on whether a finding would be important if it were true, rather than assessing whether it is true [74]. Authors value rigorous peer review [68], but the process may not always provide this.

A new phenomenon, fake peer review, is undermining the quality of published research [75]. Journals often ask prospective authors to recommend reviewers. Some individuals use the opportunity to identify fictitious reviewers whose email addresses lead back to themselves [75]. This has now expanded into 'a lucrative business practice' in which companies provide a peer review service for authors desperate for publications [75, 76]. Fake peer review is now a common reason for the retraction of papers [77, 78].

Predatory Journals and Conferences

Many journals, often with impressive titles, exist solely to make money from unsuspecting authors. Over 8,000 such journals published an estimated 420,000 papers in 2014 [79]. The journals create fake impact factors and often use titles similar to established journals, with a publisher logo modelled on a reputable organisation [80]. Most have editorial boards but the members are often fake or have had their names used without permission [81]. The journals offer rapid publication in a peer-reviewed journal, although the peer review can be lax or non-existent [80, 82].

Predatory journals take advantage of the publish or perish culture to dupe the unwary. The fee for publication is usually much lower for predatory journals (median $100) than for legitimate open access journals (median $1,865) [81]. A website of predatory journals was compiled and curated by the librarian Jeffrey Beall [83], but this has now been removed because of pressure on the librarian and his university from journals identified on the list [84]. Its successor is Cabell's Blacklist but, unlike Beall's list, a fee is charged for access [85].

These journals are considered a global threat [86, 87], providing a platform for poor quality or fabricated research, and for those with strongly held beliefs [84, 88]. Their papers are easily accessed on

Google Scholar [81], and some reputable research databases, such as Scopus and Web of Science, include journals that are suspected of being predatory [85]. How many readers interrupt their internet searches to check the credentials of papers in journals with plausible titles, and how many go on to cite such papers in their own work? Two groups have provided helpful criteria to identify predatory journals, such as poor spelling and grammar [81, 89]. The remaining challenge is to stop the activities of unscrupulous journals, or to convert them into legitimate ones [80, 89].

Another profit-driven feature of research environment is the predatory conference [90, 91]. In this, researchers are offered the opportunity to present their work at a prestigious sounding conference, in return for a substantial registration fee. The researcher can then claim to have given an invited lecture at an international conference. This is an important indicator of academic success, which can enhance the career prospects of young researchers. The downside is that it wastes time and money, as the conference may be of little interest, and sometimes the hotel room, which the conference organisers kindly offered at discounted rates, may not have been booked [90]. It seems that every facet of the research process is subject to misconduct.

CONFLICT OF INTEREST

Conflict of interest occurs when the validity of research may be compromised because the researcher stands to gain in some way from the findings of a study. Financial conflict of interest, in which researchers and clinicians are given money, research grants, shares, gifts or travel expenses, is widely recognised. The total sums involved are substantial. In the US, where the drug and medical devices companies are legally obliged to declare payment to doctors and teaching hospitals, $4.2 billion was disbursed for research in 2017, and a further $2.8 billion in general payments [92]. Non-financial conflicts of interest are less easily measured, but they refer to the way in which opportunities for career advancement and professional reputation could influence behaviour [93]. For example, some might be reluctant to criticise an influential researcher, or be unduly willing to criticise a potential rival.

Financial Conflicts

Financial conflicts of interest are common among the researchers who conduct clinical trials [94–96]. The impact of conflict of interest can be assessed by comparing the outcomes of the trials that have or do not have authors with financial conflicts. Many studies have shown what appears to be a largely consistent effect, that trials in which authors have financial conflicts are more likely to produce positive findings [94–98].

Most medical journals ask authors to disclose conflicts of interest. This is important, because it allows readers to 'discount the results of otherwise sound studies' [99]. However, financial conflicts interest are often only partially disclosed, or not disclosed at all [100, 101]. Although estimates vary across studies, over one half of authors do not fully disclose their financial conflicts of interest [101, 102]. Whether or not disclosed, these conflicts 'significantly influence whether studies report findings that are favourable to industry' [96,98].

Industry bias can also occur when trials are partly or fully funded by companies that make the drugs and medical devices being tested. One recent review reported that industry-supported trials had more favourable results and conclusions than those with other sources of funding [103]. A similar study, which focused on cardiovascular disease, found that industry-funded trials 'were almost 4 times more likely to report a positive outcome' [104].

If conflict of interest could lead to bias in trials, this will also affect the systematic reviews, which synthesise the findings of these trials. However, reviewers seldom take this into account. An assessment of 118 systematic reviews found that only 5 reported on conflict of interest among authors of the trials and none considered whether this might impact on the findings [105]. In two similar studies, the proportions of systematic reviews that addressed conflict of interest were 0% and 6.9% [106, 107].

The authors of systematic reviews can have their own conflicts of interest. Several studies have found that financial conflict of interest is common among the authors of the systematic reviews [108–110]. This can sometimes lead to biased reporting. For example, an analysis of 26 systematic reviews of neuraminidase (for flu) showed that 88% of the reviews whose authors had financial conflicts of interest recommended the use of the drugs, compared to only 17% of reviews without conflict [111]. A recent overview of such studies reported that the interpretation was more enthusiastic and the methodological quality was poorer than in reviews with financial conflicts of interest [112]. Reporting of negative statements (about harms or lack of effectiveness) may also be influenced by conflicts of interest: among systematic reviews of antidepressants, those with industry involvement were much less likely (2%–44%) to report negative statement than non-conflicted reviews [113].

Another concern is with financial conflict of interest of editors of medical journals. Some 42% of editors of American medical journals receive payments in an average year, mainly from the pharmaceutical industry [114]. A review of 713 editors from 26 specialities found that the median payment was $11 [115], although the frequency and value of payments varied across specialties. Among editors of 5 leading journals on spine research, the median declared payment was $3,152, with 15% receiving >$10,000 [116]. In dermatology 87% of editors received payments, with the top 10 receiving over $250,000 [117]. Among surgical journals the sums received ranged from $13 to $65,595, with 70% receiving >$1,500 [118]. There is no evidence that these payments influence judgements on which manuscripts are published.

Non-Financial Conflicts

Non-financial conflicts of interest form a diverse group, which include academic associations, research interests, personal relationships, political affiliations, religious views and intellectual passions [119–121]. These interests have been described as the 'values, goals and obligations' that may arise from personal, social and professional commitments [122]. One concern is that personal and professional advantage could influence judgement about right and wrong: as Cappola and Fitzgerald put it 'the prospect of fame may be even more seductive than fortune' [123]. The hypercompetitive research environment may increase the desire for personal and profession benefit.

Researcher allegiance to a particular school of thought is another form of non-financial conflict of interest. There is 'substantial and robust' evidence that researcher allegiance to psychotherapy influenced the reported effectiveness of these treatments [124]. The systematic reviews of mammography to detect breast cancer provide another example of how the professions of the authors can influence the findings: 63% of the reviews conducted by clinicians supported mammography, whereas only 32% of reviews by non-clinicians (epidemiologists and public health specialists) did so [125]. Possibly those with the responsibility of treating patients have different beliefs from those of the methodologists.

Concern about non-financial conflicts of interest has led many medical journals to ask for authors to declare such interests [120, 121]. However there is an active debate about non-financial interests, focusing on how they are defined, whether addressing them may detract attention from financial conflicts, and if declarations could have unintended consequences [126–128]. As is commonly the case, the argument would be resolved if there were 'better empirical evidence about the prevalence and influence of non-financial interests' [93].

INDIVIDUAL LEVEL EXPLANATIONS FOR RESEARCH MISCONDUCT

Research misconduct is committed by individuals, and it would be easy to conclude that they should be punished. But to prevent misdeeds, a deeper understanding of the individual's motivation is required. This section, and the next, explore the factors underlying research misconduct.

Data Fabrication and the Dark Triad

Major data fraud is most likely the result of personality disorder. Research from psychology suggests that the Dark Triad of personality traits (narcissism, Machiavellianism and psychopathy) are associated with deceit and wrongdoing [129]. Narcissism is associated with vanity and the need for admiration, and with a sense of superiority and entitlement. Machiavellian individuals are cunning, and manipulate and exploit with a cynical disregard for morality.

Psychopathy is the tendency for impulsive, thrill-seeking and antisocial behaviour, accompanied by callousness and lack of remorse [130]. These traits may explain why some individuals fabricate data on a large scale, and can do so many times. Such fraud is a rare event, but preventing it would be challenging because this would involve changing attributes of personality. Vigilance in fraud detection to minimise its consequences would be a more realistic approach.

The Fraud Triangle, Data Falsification and Questionable Research Practices

The fraud triangle provides a helpful model of the causes of data falsification and questionable research practices. It has been widely used in business and accounting to identify and understand financial misconduct [131, 132]. It has also been used to investigate cheating behaviour in students [133, 134] and has recently been used to assess research misconduct [135].

The model identifies three explanatory factors: incentives, opportunity and rationalisation. In research these correspond to the perverse incentives that encourage misbehaviour; the opportunities provided by flexibility in the design, conduct and analysis of research, and an oversight system based mainly on trust; and the rationalisation that occurs through the psychological factors that enable researchers to engage in questionable research practices. The incentives are considerable: career advancement, financial reward, (misplaced) respect from peers and invitations to speak at international conferences. The opportunities arise because individual researchers usually have complete control of the conduct and analysis of studies, with few checks on whether correct procedures are followed. The ability to rationalise misconduct is an inherent weakness of honest people.

HOW HONEST PEOPLE RATIONALISE MISCONDUCT

Most people think of themselves as honest [136], but dishonest behaviour is a worldwide problem [137]. Scientists are motivated by curiosity, a search for knowledge, and by the recognition and esteem of colleagues [138, 139]; but some can deviate from the highest standards of behaviour. This section reviews how societal and individual factors interact to influence misbehaviour. It does not suggest that all, or even the majority, of researchers engage in misbehaviour, but rather explores how some may be drawn into misconduct.

Societal Factors

The extent to which individuals engage in dishonest behaviour depends on the moral values of their culture [140]. Dishonesty is much more common in weak institutions with cultural values that permit rule violations. In such circumstances cheating becomes infectious: 'seeing someone else cheat without apparent consequences strongly encourages others to cheat' [141]. This could be because they believe that other people benefit from cheating and they will be disadvantaged if they do not do it [142]. Another factor is the sense of fairness in the research process [143]. If researchers perceive that they are being unfairly treated (e.g. by funding bodies, ethical review boards and the peer review system) they are more likely to engage in questionable research practices [144]. Individuals are able to reinterpret their behaviour in a self-serving manner [136, 145], a process that is exacerbated by 'conditions of extreme competition [which] lead to unethical behaviour' [146].

Cognitive Biases

Psychologists have identified many types of cognitive bias that influence behaviour. The problem with these biases is that researchers are usually unaware of them, so that even careful self-examination will not identify them [147]. There is good evidence that unconscious bias influences clinical reasoning [148, 149] and could subvert clinical evidence [150]. Most researchers do not deliberately set out to manipulate, but rather unconscious biases allow them to do so. Four cognitive biases most relevant to research studies are discussed.

Blind Spot Bias

A curious thing about people is that most think they are objective, while recognising that others may be prone to bias [147, 151]. This is blind spot bias. It could explain why clinicians and researchers accept gifts from the pharmaceutical industry, because they believe they are immune to their effects [152]. In fact, receipt of a gift induces a sense of obligation and the need to reciprocate [153, 154]. Individuals may think they can take the money because they will not be biased, when in reality accepting a gift often influences judgement in favour of the giver. The susceptibility of people to this bias could help explain why the drug and medical devices industries give away money and gifts so freely: they are confident of a return on their investment [153].

Confirmation Bias

Confirmation bias describes the unconscious desire to make reality conform to a prior belief [155]. Possibly this bias could encourage researchers to 'fudge data or their analysis to support their preconceived beliefs' [156]. For example, a potential confounder might be included in an analysis only if this resulted in a statistically significant result [157]. This bias can influence the interpretation of study findings [150], so that conclusions fit with what people wish to be true [158]. Thus, a strong belief in the effectiveness of the treatment could lead the researcher to replace the pre-specified outcome measure, if it did not support that belief, with another that showed the treatment to be beneficial. Gorman has speculated that 'the freedom to pick and choose which results to publish' could explain the high frequency of effective treatments in the field of drug misuse [159]. Finally, Goodyear-Smith and colleagues have suggested that strongly held views may have influenced the inclusion and exclusion of trials in a systematic review, to ensure that a desired conclusion was reached [160].

Optimism Bias

People also have a remarkable tendency to think that future events will turn out well [161]. This is optimism bias, the difference between hopeful expectation and harsh reality [162]. An example is an unwarranted belief in the effectiveness of a new treatment. Researchers designing trials usually overestimate the amount of benefit that patients will experience, so that their sample size calculations lead to studies being too small to detect important treatment benefits [163, 164]. Optimism bias may also explain why recruitment to clinical trials is poor. This is enshrined in Lasagna's Law of patient recruitment, which holds that 'the number of patients who are actually available for a trial is about one tenth to one third of what was originally estimated' [165]. In consequence, many trials recruit fewer patients than intended, and some are abandoned because recruitment is so poor.

Hindsight Bias

Hindsight bias is the name given to the phenomenon of being wise after the event [166]. Sometimes, when an unexpected finding emerges from an analysis, hindsight bias can lead a researcher to think that they 'knew it all along' [167]. Memory can be distorted to the extent that the person misremembers having predicted exactly that result. This could explain why data torturing is problematic. Multiple analyses and subgroup analyses are conducted until a significant result is obtained; with hindsight bias this becomes a predicted finding. It then becomes perfectly acceptable to present the serendipitous result as a pre-specified hypothesis. In the process, people may congratulate themselves on their insight and ability to predict.

Moral Licensing

Most individuals believe they are honest and would resist committing dishonest acts [136]. Moral licensing can change this: it suggests that 'acting virtuously can subsequently free people to act less-than-virtuously' [168]. This may occur because previous virtuous acts establish an individual's moral self-worth, which is not threatened by a subsequent immoral act [169]. Even planning to do good in the future enables people to misbehave today [168]. This mechanism would allow individuals to falsify data or manipulate their analyses, so long they had a sufficient store of virtue, and the degree of misconduct did not threaten their sense of moral self-worth.

Motivation for Research

Undertaking a research study, such as a clinical trial, requires great energy and enthusiasm. Few people would decide to spend several years designing and conducting a clinical trial, if they did not think that the treatment was likely to be effective. Further, to obtain funding for a trial the researchers need to make a convincing case that the treatment is likely to be beneficial. The effort required to run a trial can create a desire to obtain a particular result, which affects judgement [158], and could lead to research misconduct [170]. The thinking may go along the lines of: 'I've worked so hard on this, and I know this works, and I need to get this publication' [170]. During the analysis some researchers may search for proof of effectiveness of a treatment by conducting several different analyses, or deleting data points that clearly do not fit the expected pattern. In many instances, this search may be well intentioned, but it has a problem; distorting the analysis to fit a prior belief invalidates the eventual finding

DISCUSSION

This chapter has reviewed possible causes of research misconduct, and could give the impression that a majority of researchers engage in misbehaviour. This would be wrong. Most researchers are honest and strive to conduct high quality studies. The rare instances of major fraud are perpetrated by a few dishonest individuals [171]. But malpractice in research is a wider concern, with 'many shades of grey along the spectrum that runs from integrity to research misconduct' [172]. Rather than just focusing on the infamous individuals, efforts should also address 'the health of the orchard, not just the bad apples in it' [173]. Questionable research practices, which are engaged in by a minority of scientists, are sufficiently common that they present a serious problem [173]. The causes of both major and minor acts of data fabrication and manipulation need to be understood so that appropriate strategies can be put in place to minimise their effects.

Perverse incentives provide part of the explanation for misconduct. Fierce competition for jobs and for research funding occurs in an environment that places a very high value on excellence. This can lead a few to manipulate their studies to produce statistically and clinically significant findings. The current emphasis on excellence, as Moore and colleagues concluded, is 'a pernicious and dangerous rhetoric that undermines the very foundations of good research and scholarship' [11].

The method of research oversight, peer review, is based on trust, with researchers believing they have a very low risk of their misconduct being detected [174]. As cheating can be infectious [141], there is the risk that 'the scientific enterprise itself becomes inherently corrupt' [3]. An objective observer might well conclude that the research system was designed to promote research misconduct.

The fraud triangle provides a helpful model to explain the common forms of research misconduct. The research environment provides strong incentives for misconduct. The opportunities for misbehaviour stem from the lax system of oversight and the flexibilities inherent in the conduct of research. Finally, the ability of humans to rationalise their behaviour, through cognitive biases, enables honest individuals to behave dishonestly. An important point about the fraud model is that it clarifies how behaviours carried out by individuals are to a large extent driven by the research environment. This suggests that substantial changes to the incentive system and the methods of research oversight will be needed to prevent study manipulation and to ensure that cheating is detected not rewarded.

This book has reviewed the nature, extent and causes of misconduct and poor quality research. Appendix 1 summarises the findings and Appendix 2 reviews a range of initiatives that have been proposed to address the common failings in research. The next chapter outlines how an overarching strategy to improve the quality of medical research could be developed.

REFERENCES

1. Kamerlin, S.C. (2015). Hypercompetition in biomedical research evaluation and its impact on young scientist careers. *Int. Microbiol.* 18: 253–261.

2. Joynson, C. and Leyser, O. (2015). The culture of scientific research. *F1000Res.* https://doi.org/10.12688/f1000research.6163.1.

3. Edwards, M.A. and Roy, S. (2017). Academic research in the 21st century: maintaining scientific integrity in a climate of perverse incentives and hypercompetition. *Environ. Eng. Sci.* 34: 51–61.

4. Woolston, C. (2018). Satisfaction in science. *Nature* 562: 611–614.

5. Chubb, J. and Watermeyer, R. (2017). Artifice or integrity in the marketization of research impact? Investigating the moral economy of (pathways to) impact statements within research funding proposals in the UK and Australia. *Stud. High. Educ.* 42: 2360–2372.

6. Moher, D., Naudet, F., Cristea, I.A. et al. (2018). Assessing scientists for hiring, promotion, and tenure. *PLoS Biol.* https://doi.org/10.1371/journal.pbio.2004089.

7. McKiernan, E.C., Schimanski, L.A., Munoz Nieves, C. et al. (2019). *elife* https://doi.org/10.7554/eLife.47338.

8. Tijdink, J.K., Verbeke, R., and Smulders, Y.M. (2014). Publication pressure and scientific misconduct in medical scientists. *J. Empir. Res. Hum. Res. Ethics* 9: 64–71.

9. Casadevall, A. and Fang, F.C. (2014). Causes for the persistence of impact factor mania. *MBio* https://doi.org/10.1128/mBio.01342-14.

10. Haven, T.L., Bouter, L.M., Smulders, Y.M. et al. (2019). Perceived publication pressure in Amsterdam: survey of all disciplinary fields and academic ranks. *PLoS One* https://doi.org/10.1371/journal.pone.0217931.

11. Moore, S., Neylon, C., Eve, M.P. et al. (2017). "Excellence R us": university research and the fetishisation of excellence. *Palgrave Commun.* https://doi.org/10.1057/palcomms.2016.105.

12. Fang, F.C. and Casadevall, A. (2015). Competitive science: is competition ruining science? *Infect. Immun.* 83: 1229–1233.

13. Anderson, M.S., Ronning, E.A., De Vries, R. et al. (2007). The perverse effects of competition on scientists' work and relationships. *Sci. Eng. Ethics* 13: 437–461.

14. Casadevall, A. (2019). Duke University's huge misconduct fine is a reminder to reward rigour. *Nature* 568: 7.

15. Nosek, B.A., Spies, J.R., and Motyl, M. (2012). Scientific Utopia: II. Restructuring incentives and practices to promote truth over Publishability. *Perspect. Psychol. Sci.* 7: 615–631.

16. Ware, J.J. and Munafo, M.R. (2015). Significance chasing in research practice: causes, consequences and possible solutions. *Addiction* 110: 4–8.

17. Wager, E., Williams, P. et al. (2013). *BMJ* https://doi.org/10.1136/bmj.f5248.

18. Zietman, A.L. (2017). The ethics of scientific publishing: black, white, and "fifty shades of gray". *Int. J. Radiat. Oncol. Biol. Phys.* 99: 275–279.

19. Ten Hagen, K.G. (2016). Novel or reproducible: that is the question. *Glycobiology* https://doi.org/10.1093/glycob/cww036.

20. Millar, N., Salager-Meyer, F., Budgell, B. et al. (2019). *Engl. Specif. Purp.* 54: 139–151.

21. Reich, E.S. (2013). Science publishing: the golden club. *Nature* 502: 291–293.

22. Schmid, S.L. (2017). Five years post-DORA: promoting best practices for research assessment. *Mol. Biol. Cell* 28: 2941–2944.

23. Paulus, F.M., Cruz, N., and Krach, S. (2018). The impact factor fallacy. *Front. Psychol.* https://doi.org/10.3389/fpsyg.2018.01487.

24. Zhang, L., Rousseau, R., and Sivertsen, G. (2017). Science deserves to be judged by its contents, not by its wrapping: revisiting Seglen's work on journal impact and research evaluation. *PLoS One* https://doi.org/10.1371/journal.pone.0174205.

25. Chapman, C.A., Bicca-Marques, J.C., Calvignac-Spencer, S. et al. (2019). Games academics play and their consequences: how authorship, h-index and journal impact factors are shaping the future of academia. *Proc. Biol. Sci.* https://doi.org/10.1098/rspb.2019.2047.

26. Martin, B.R. (2016). Editors' JIF-boosting stratagems – which are appropriate and which not? *Res. Policy* 45: 1–7.

27. Ioannidis, J.P.A. and Thombs, B.D. (2019). A user's guide to inflated and manipulated impact factors. *Eur. J. Clin. Investig.* https://doi.org/10.1111/eci.13151.

28. Grimes, D.R., Bauch, C.T., and Ioannidis, J.P.A. (2018). Modelling science trustworthiness under publish or perish pressure. *R. Soc. Open Sci.* https://doi.org/10.1098/rsos.171511.

29. Eshre, C.W.G. (2018). Protect us from poor-quality medical research. *Hum. Reprod.* 33: 770–776.

30. Smaldino, P.E. and McElreath, R. (2016). The natural selection of bad science. *R. Soc. Open Sci.* https://doi.org/10.1098/rsos.160384.

31. Malicki, M. and Marusic, A. (2014). Is there a solution to publication bias? Researchers call for changes in dissemination of clinical research results. *J. Clin. Epidemiol.* 67: 1103–1110.

32. Berendt, L., Petersen, L.G., Bach, K.F. et al. (2017). Barriers towards the publication of academic drug trials. Follow-up of trials approved by the Danish medicines agency. *PLoS One* https://doi.org/10.1371/journal.pone.0172581.

33. Song, F., Loke, Y., and Hooper, L. (2014). Why are medical and health-related studies not being published? A systematic review of reasons given by investigators. *PLoS One* https://doi.org/10.1371/journal.pone.0110418.

34. Abritis, A. and McCook, A. (2017). Cash incentives for papers go global. *Science* 357: 541.

35. Breet, E., Botha, J., Horn, L. et al. (2018). Academic and scientific authorship practices: a survey among south African researchers. *J. Empir. Res. Hum. Res. Ethics* 13: 412–420.

36. Guraya, S.Y., Norman, R.I., Khoshhal, K.I. et al. (2016). Publish or perish mantra in the medical field: a systematic review of the reasons, consequences and remedies. *Pak. J. Med. Sci.* 32: 1562–1567.

37. Merton, R.K. (1968). The Matthew effect in science: the reward and communication systems of science are considered. *Science* 159: 56–63.

38. Oravec, J.A. (2017). The manipulation of scholarly rating and measurement systems: constructing excellence in an era of academic stardom. *Teach. High. Educ.* 22: 423–436.

39. Werner, R. (2015). The focus on bibliometrics makes papers less useful. *Nature* 517: 245.

40. Frost, J. and Brockmann, J. (2014). When qualitative productivity is equated with quantitative productivity: scholars caught in a performance paradox. *Zeitschrift Fur Erziehungswissenschaft* 17: 25–45.

41. Fire, M. and Guestrin, C. (2019). Over-optimization of academic publishing metrics: observing Goodhart's law in action. *GigaScience* https://doi.org/10.1093/gigascience/giz053.

42. Ebrahim, N., Salehi, H., Ma, E. et al. (2013). Effective strategies for increasing citation frequency. *Int. Educ. Stud.* 6: 93–99.

43. Buela-Casal, G. (2014). Pathological publishing: a new psychological disorder with legal consequences? *Eur. J. Psychol. Appl.Legal Context* 6: 91–97.

44. Ioannidis, J.P. (2015). A generalized view of self-citation: direct, co-author, collaborative, and coercive induced self-citation. *J. Psychosom. Res.* 78: 7–11.

45. Seeber, M., Cattaneo, M., Meoli, M. et al. (2019). Self-citations as strategic response to the use of metrics for career decisions. *Res. Policy* 48: 478–491.

46. Biagioli, M. (2016). Watch out for cheats in citation game. *Nature* 535: 201.

47. Li, W.H., Aste, T., Caccioli, F. et al. (2019). Reciprocity and impact in academic careers. *Epj Data Sci.* https://doi.org/10.1140/epjds/s13688-019-0199-3.

48. Thombs, B.D., Levis, A.W., Razykov, I. et al. (2015). Potentially coercive self-citation by peer reviewers: a cross-sectional study. *J. Psychosom. Res.* 78: 1–6.

49. Van Noorden, R. (2020). Highly cited researcher banned from journal board for citation abuse. *Nature* 578: 200–201.

50. Martin, B.R. (2013). Whither research integrity? Plagiarism, self-plagiarism and coercive citation in an age of research assessment. *Res. Policy* 42: 1005–1014.

51. Wallace, M.B., Bowman, D., Hamilton-Gibbs, H. et al. (2018). Ethics in publication, part 2: duplicate publishing, salami slicing, and large retrospective multicenter case series. *Endoscopy* 50: 463–465.

52. Ebrahim, S., Montoya, L., Kamal El Din, M. et al. (2016). Randomized trials are frequently fragmented in multiple secondary publications. *J. Clin. Epidemiol.* 79: 130–139.

53. Madsen, R.R. (2019). Scientific impact and the quest for visibility. *FEBS J.* 286: 3968–3974.

54. Glasziou, P., Sanders, S., and Hoffmann, T. (2020). Waste in covid-19 research. *BMJ* https://doi.org/10.1136/bmj.m1847.

55. Higginson, A.D. and Munafo, M.R. (2016). Current incentives for scientists lead to underpowered studies with erroneous conclusions. *PLoS Biol.* https://doi.org/10.1371/journal.pbio.1002106.

56. Alberts, B. and Shine, K. (1994). Scientists and the integrity of research. *Science* 266: 1660–1661.

57. Sztompka, P. et al. (2007). *J. Class. Sociol.* 7: 211–220.

58. Wallach, J.D., Gonsalves, G.S., and Ross, J.S. (2018). Research, regulatory, and clinical decision-making: the importance of scientific integrity. *J. Clin. Epidemiol.* 93: 88–93.

59. Schechter, A.N., Wyngaarden, J.B., Edsall, J.T. et al. (1989). Colloquium on scientific authorship – rights and responsibilities. *FASEB J.* 3: 209–217.

60. Smith, R. (2006). Research misconduct: the poisoning of the well. *J. R. Soc. Med.* 99: 232–237.

61. Kornfeld, D.S. (2012). Perspective: research misconduct: the search for a remedy. *Acad. Med.* 87: 877–882.

62. Kornfeld, D.S. and Titus, S.L. (2016). Stop ignoring misconduct. *Nature* 537: 29–30.

63. McNutt, M. and Nerem, R.M. (2017). Research integrity revisited. *Science* 356: 115.

64. Gunsalus, C.K., McNutt, M.K., Martinson, B.C. et al. (2019). Overdue: a US advisory board for research integrity. *Nature* 566: 173–175.

65. Moore, R.A., Derry, S., and McQuay, H.J. (2010). Fraud or flawed: adverse impact of fabricated or poor quality research. *Anaesthesia* 65: 327–330.

66. Horbach, S. and Halffman, W.W. (2018). The changing forms and expectations of peer review. *Res. Integr. Peer Rev.* https://doi.org/10.1186/s41073-018-0051-5.

67. Chauvin, A., Ravaud, P., Baron, G. et al. (2015). The most important tasks for peer reviewers evaluating a randomized controlled trial are not congruent with the tasks most often requested by journal editors. *BMC Med.* https://doi.org/10.1186/s12916-015-0395-3.

68. Hames, I. (2014). Peer review at the beginning of the 21st century. *Sci. Ed.* 1: 4–8.

69. Nagler, A., Ovitsh, R., Dumenco, L. et al. (2019). Communities of practice in peer review: outlining a group review process. *Acad. Med.* 94: 1437–1442.

70. Heneghan, C. and McCartney, M. (2019). Declaring interests and restoring trust in medicine. *BMJ* https://doi.org/10.1136/bmj.d7202.

71. Bruce, R., Chauvin, A., Trinquart, L. et al. (2016). Impact of interventions to improve the quality of peer review of biomedical journals: a systematic review and meta-analysis. *BMC Med.* https://doi.org/10.1186/s12916-016-0631-5.

72. Moher, D. and Altman, D.G. (2015). Four proposals to help improve the medical research literature. *PLoS Med.* https://doi.org/10.1371/journal.pmed.1001864.

73. Patel, J. (2014). Why training and specialization is needed for peer review: a case study of peer review for randomized controlled trials. *BMC Med.* https://doi.org/10.1186/s12916-014-0128-z.

74. Kaelin, W.G. Jr. (2017). Publish houses of brick, not mansions of straw. *Nature* 545: 387.

75. Haug, C.J. (2015). Peer-review fraud – hacking the scientific publication process. *N. Engl. J. Med.* 373: 2393–2395.

76. Barbour, V. (2015). Perverse incentives and perverse publishing practices. *Sci. Bull.* 60: 1225–1226.

77. Campos-Varela, I., Ruano-Ravina, A. et al. (2018). *Gac. Sanit.* https://doi.org/10.1016/j.gaceta.2018.01.009.

78. Moylan, E.C. and Kowalczuk, M.K. (2016). Why articles are retracted: a retrospective cross-sectional study of retraction notices at BioMed central. *BMJ Open* https://doi.org/10.1136/bmjopen-2016-012047.

79. Shen, C., Bjork, B.C. et al. (2015). *BMC Med.* https://doi.org/10.1186/s12916-015-0469-2.

80. Moher, D. and Moher, E. (2016). Stop predatory publishers now: act collaboratively. *Ann. Intern. Med.* 164: 616–617.

81. Shamseer, L., Moher, D., Maduekwe, O. et al. (2017). Potential predatory and legitimate biomedical journals: can you tell the difference? A cross-sectional comparison. *BMC Med.* https://doi.org/10.1186/s12916-017-0785-9.

82. Sorokowski, P., Kulczycki, E., Sorokowska, A. et al. (2017). Predatory journals recruit fake editor. *Nature* 543: 481–483.

83. Beall, J. (2012). Predatory publishers are corrupting open access. *Nature* 489: 179.

84. Beall, J. (2017). What I learned from predatory publishers. *Biochem Med.* 27: 273–278.

85. Strielkowski, W. (2018). Predatory publishing: what are the alternatives to Beall's list? *Am. J. Med.* 131: 333–334.

86. Grudniewicz, A., Moher, D., Cobey, K.D. et al. (2019). Predatory journals: no definition, no defence. *Nature* 576: 210–212.

87. Sharma, H. and Verma, S. (2018). Predatory journals: the rise of worthless biomedical science. *J. Postgrad. Med.* 64: 226–231.

88. Rupp, M., Anastasopoulou, L., Wintermeyer, E. et al. (2019). Predatory journals: a major threat in orthopaedic research. *Int. Orthop.* 43: 509–517.

89. Laine, C. and Winker, M.A. (2017). Identifying predatory or pseudo-journals. *Biochem Med.* 27: 285–291.

90. Cress, P.E. (2017). Are predatory conferences the dark side of the open access movement? *Aesthet. Surg. J.* 37: 734–738.

91. Collins, E.M. and Bassat, Q. (2018). The scientific integrity of journal publications in the age of 'Fake News'. *J. Trop. Pediatr.* 64: 360–363.

92. Ross, J.S. et al. (2019). *BMJ* https://doi.org/10.1136/bmj.l1379.

93. Saver, R.S. (2012). Is it really all about the money? Reconsidering non-financial interests in medical research. *J. Law Med. Ethics* 40: 467–481.

94. Ahn, R., Woodbridge, A., Abraham, A. et al. (2017). Financial ties of principal investigators and randomized controlled trial outcomes: cross sectional study. *BMJ* https://doi.org/10.1136/bmj.i6770.

95. Riaz, H., Khan, M.S., Riaz, I.B. et al. (2016). Conflicts of interest and outcomes of cardiovascular trials. *Am. J. Cardiol.* 117: 858–860.

96. Cherla, D.V., Viso, C.P., Olavarria, O.A. et al. (2018). The impact of financial conflict of interest on surgical research: an observational study of published manuscripts. *World J. Surg.* 42: 2757–2762.

97. Lopez, J., Lopez, S., Means, J. et al. (2015). Financial conflicts of interest: an association between funding and findings in

plastic surgery. *Plast. Reconstr. Surg.* https://doi.org/10.1097/PRS.0000000000001718.

98. Cherla, D.V., Viso, C.P., Holihan, J.L. et al. (2019). The effect of financial conflict of interest, disclosure status, and relevance on medical research from the United States. *J. Gen. Intern. Med.* 34: 429–434.

99. Loder, E., Brizzell, C., and Godlee, F. (2015). Revisiting the commercial-academic interface in medical journals. *BMJ* https://doi.org/10.1136/bmj.h2957.

100. Bauchner, H., Fontanarosa, P.B., Flanagin, A. et al. (2018). *JAMA* 320: 2315–2318.

101. Cherla, D.V., Olavarria, O.A., Holihan, J.L. et al. (2017). Discordance of conflict of interest self-disclosure and the centers of Medicare and Medicaid services. *J. Surg. Res.* 218: 18–22.

102. Dunn, A.G., Coiera, E., Mandl, K.D. et al. (2016). Conflict of interest disclosure in biomedical research: a review of current practices, biases, and the role of public registries in improving transparency. *Res. Integr. Peer Rev.* https://doi.org/10.1186/s41073-016-0006-7.

103. Lundh, A., Lexchin, J., Mintzes, B. et al. (2018). Industry sponsorship and research outcome: systematic review with meta-analysis. *Intensive Care Med.* 44: 1603–1612.

104. Riaz, H., Raza, S., Khan, M.S. et al. (2015). Impact of funding source on clinical trial results including cardiovascular outcome trials. *Am. J. Cardiol.* 116: 1944–1947.

105. Elia, N., von Elm, E., Chatagner, A. et al. (2016). How do authors of systematic reviews deal with research malpractice and misconduct in original studies? A cross-sectional analysis of systematic reviews and survey of their authors. *BMJ Open* https://doi.org/10.1136/bmjopen-2015-010442.

106. Faggion, C.M. Jr., Monje, A., and Wasiak, J. (2018). Appraisal of systematic reviews on the management of peri-implant diseases with two methodological tools. *J. Clin. Periodontol.* 45: 754–766.

107. Benea, C., Turner, K.A., Roseman, M. et al. (2020). Reporting of financial conflicts of interest in meta-analyses of drug trials published in high-impact medical journals: comparison of results

from 2017 to 2018 and 2009. *Syst. Rev.* https://doi.org/10.1186/s13643-020-01318-5.

108. Hakoum, M.B., Anouti, S., Al-Gibbawi, M. et al. (2016). Reporting of financial and non-financial conflicts of interest by authors of systematic reviews: a methodological survey. *BMJ Open* https://doi.org/10.1136/bmjopen-2016-011997.

109. Bou-Karroum, L., Hakoum, M.B., Hammoud, M.Z. et al. (2018). Reporting of financial and non-financial conflicts of interest in systematic reviews on health policy and systems research: a cross sectional survey. *Int. J. Health Policy Manag.* 7: 711–717.

110. Lieb, K., von der Osten-Sacken, J., Stoffers-Winterling, J. et al. (2016). Conflicts of interest and spin in reviews of psychological therapies: a systematic review. *BMJ Open* https://doi.org/10.1136/bmjopen-2015-010606.

111. Dunn, A.G., Arachi, D., Hudgins, J. et al. (2014). Financial conflicts of interest and conclusions about neuraminidase inhibitors for influenza: an analysis of systematic reviews. *Ann. Intern. Med.* 161: 513–518.

112. Hansen, C., Lundh, A., Rasmussen, K. et al. (2019). Financial conflicts of interest in systematic reviews: associations with results, conclusions, and methodological quality. *Cochrane Database Syst. Rev.* https://doi.org/10.1002/14651858.MR000047.pub2.

113. Ebrahim, S., Bance, S., Athale, A. et al. (2016). Meta-analyses with industry involvement are massively published and report no caveats for antidepressants. *J. Clin. Epidemiol.* 70: 155–163.

114. Wong, V.S.S., Avalos, L.N., and Callaham, M.L. (2019). Industry payments to physician journal editors. *PLoS One* https://doi.org/10.1371/journal.pone.0211495.

115. Liu, J.J., Bell, C.M., Matelski, J.J. et al. (2017). Payments by US pharmaceutical and medical device manufacturers to US medical journal editors: retrospective observational study. *BMJ* https://doi.org/10.1136/bmj.j4619.

116. Janssen, S.J., Bredenoord, A.L., Dhert, W. et al. (2015). Potential conflicts of interest of editorial board members from five leading spine journals. *PLoS One* https://doi.org/10.1371/journal.pone.0127362.

117. Updyke, K.M., Niu, W., St Claire, C. et al. (2018). Editorial boards of dermatology journals and their potential financial conflict of interest. *Dermatol. Online J.*

118. Alexander, H. (2019). Industry payments received by the editors of the top 100 surgery journals. *Aesthet. Surg. J.* https://doi.org/10.1093/asj/sjz059.

119. Bion, J., Antonelli, M., Blanch, L. et al. (2018). White paper: statement on conflicts of interest. *Intensive Care Med.* 44: 1657–1668.

120. Shawwa, K., Kallas, R., Koujanian, S. et al. (2016). Requirements of clinical journals for Authors' disclosure of financial and non-financial conflicts of interest: a cross sectional study. *PLoS One* https://doi.org/10.1371/journal.pone.0152301.

121. Khamis, A.M., Hakoum, M.B., Bou-Karroum, L. et al. (2017). Requirements of health policy and services journals for authors to disclose financial and non-financial conflicts of interest: a cross-sectional study. *Health Res. Policy Syst.* https://doi.org/10.1186/s12961-017-0244-2.

122. Wiersma, M., Kerridge, I., and Lipworth, W. (2018). Dangers of neglecting non-financial conflicts of interest in health and medicine. *J. Med. Ethics* 44: 319–322.

123. Cappola, A.R. and FitzGerald, G.A. (2015). Confluence, not conflict of interest: name change necessary. *JAMA* 314: 1791–1792.

124. Munder, T., Brutsch, O., Leonhart, R. et al. (2013). Researcher allegiance in psychotherapy outcome research: an overview of reviews. *Clin. Psychol. Rev.* 33: 501–511.

125. Raichand, S., Dunn, A.G., Ong, M.S. et al. (2017). Conclusions in systematic reviews of mammography for breast cancer screening and associations with review design and author characteristics. *Syst. Rev.* https://doi.org/10.1186/s13643-017-0495-6.

126. Bero, L.A. and Grundy, Q. (2016). Why having a (nonfinancial) interest is not a conflict of interest. *PLoS Biol.* https://doi.org/10.1371/journal.pbio.2001221.

127. Wiersma, M., Kerridge, I., Lipworth, W. et al. (2018). Should we try to manage non-financial interests? *BMJ* https://doi.org/10.1136/bmj.d40.

128. Grundy, Q., Mayes, C., Holloway, K. et al. (2020). Conflict of interest as ethical shorthand: understanding the range and nature of "non-financial conflict of interest" in biomedicine. *J. Clin. Epidemiol.* 120: 1–7.

129. Jones, D.N. and Paulhus, D.L. (2017). Duplicity among the dark triad: three faces of deceit. *J. Pers. Soc. Psychol.* 113: 329–342.

130. Rauthmann, J.F. (2012). The dark triad and interpersonal perception: similarities and differences in the social consequences of narcissism, Machiavellianism, and psychopathy. *Soc. Psychol. Personal. Sci.* 3: 487–496.

131. Huang, S.Y., Lin, C.C., Chiu, A.A. et al. (2017). Fraud detection using fraud triangle risk factors. *Inf. Syst. Front.* 19: 1343–1356.

132. Raval, V. (2018). A disposition-based fraud model: theoretical integration and research agenda. *J. Bus. Ethics* 150: 741–763.

133. Choo, F. and Tan, K. (2008). The effect of fraud triangle factors on Students' cheating behaviors. *Adv. Account. Educ.* 9: 205–220.

134. MacGregor, J. and Stuebs, M. (2012). To cheat or not to cheat: rationalizing academic impropriety. *Acc. Educ.* 21: 265–287.

135. Ariail, D.L. and Crumbley, D.L. (2016). Fraud triangle and ethical leadership perspectives on detecting and preventing academic research misconduct. *J. Forensic Investig. Account.* 8: 480–500.

136. Mazar, N., Amir, O., and Ariely, D. (2008). The dishonesty of honest people: a theory of self-concept maintenance. *J. Mark. Res.* 45: 633–644.

137. Gerlach, P., Teodorescu, K., and Hertwig, R. (2019). The truth about lies: a meta-analysis on dishonest behavior. *Psychol. Bull.* 145: 1–44.

138. Lam, A. (2011). What motivates academic scientists to engage in research commercialization: 'Gold', 'ribbon' or 'puzzle'? *Res. Policy* 40: 1354–1368.

139. Franck, G. (2015). The wage of fame: how non-epistemic motives have enabled the phenomenal success of modern science. *Gerontology* 61: 89–94.

140. Gachter, S. and Schulz, J.F. (2016). Intrinsic honesty and the prevalence of rule violations across societies. *Nature* 531: 496–499.

141. Fang, F., Casadeval, A. et al. (2013). *Sci. Am. Mind* 24: 31–37.

142. Sacco, D.F., Bruton, S.V., and Brown, M. (2018). In defense of the questionable: defining the basis of research scientists' engagement in questionable research practices. *J. Empir. Res. Hum. Res. Ethics* 13: 101–110.

143. Martinson, B.C., Crain, A.L., De Vries, R. et al. (2010). The importance of organizational justice in ensuring research integrity. *J. Empir. Res. Hum. Res. Ethics* 5: 67–83.

144. Martinson, B.C., Anderson, M.S., Crain, A.L. et al. (2006). Scientists' perceptions of organizational justice and self-reported misbehaviors. *J. Empir. Res. Hum. Res. Ethics* 1: 51–66.

145. Dahl, G.B. and Ransom, M.R. (1999). Does where you stand depend on where you sit? Tithing donations and self-sewing beliefs. *Am. Econ. Rev.* 89: 703–727.

146. Rick, S. and Loewenstein, G. (2008). Commentaries and rejoinder to "the dishonesty of honest people". *J. Mark. Res.* 45: 645–648.

147. Ehrlinger, J., Gilovich, T., and Ross, L. (2005). Peering into the bias blind spot: people's assessments of bias in themselves and others. *Personal. Soc. Psychol. Bull.* 31: 680–692.

148. Saposnik, G., Redelmeier, D., Ruff, C.C. et al. (2016). Cognitive biases associated with medical decisions: a systematic review. *BMC Med. Inform Decis. Mak.* https://doi.org/10.1186/s12911-016-0377-1.

149. Blumenthal-Barby, J.S. and Krieger, H. (2015). Cognitive biases and heuristics in medical decision making: a critical review using a systematic search strategy. *Med. Decis. Mak.* 35: 539–557.

150. Seshia, S.S., Makhinson, M., and Young, G.B. (2016). 'Cognitive biases plus': covert subverters of healthcare evidence. *Evid. Based Med.* 21: 41–45.

151. Pronin, E. (2007). Perception and misperception of bias in human judgment. *Trends Cogn. Sci.* 11: 37–43.

152. Sah, S. (2012). Conflicts of interest and your physician: psychological processes that cause unexpected changes in behavior. *J. Law Med. Ethics* 40: 482–487.

153. Sah, S. and Fugh-Berman, A. (2013). Physicians under the influence: social psychology and industry marketing strategies. *J. Law Med. Ethics* 41: 665–672.

154. Katz, D., Caplan, A.L., and Merz, J.F. (2010). All gifts large and small: toward an understanding of the ethics of pharmaceutical industry gift-giving. *Am. J. Bioeth.* 10: 11–17.

155. Montibeller, G. and von Winterfeldt, D. (2015). Cognitive and motivational biases in decision and risk analysis. *Risk Anal.* 35: 1230–1251.

156. Baddeley, M. (2015). Herding, social influences and behavioural bias in scientific research: simple awareness of the hidden pressures and beliefs that influence our thinking can help to preserve objectivity. *EMBO Rep.* 16: 902–905.

157. Motulsky, H.J. (2015). Common misconceptions about data analysis and statistics. *Pharmacol. Res. Perspect.* 3: 200–205.

158. Bastardi, A., Uhlmann, E.L., and Ross, L. (2011). Wishful thinking: belief, desire, and the motivated evaluation of scientific evidence. *Psychol. Sci.* 22: 731–732.

159. Gorman, D.M. (2015). 'Everything works': the need to address confirmation bias in evaluations of drug misuse prevention interventions for adolescents. *Addiction* 110: 1539–1540.

160. Goodyear-Smith, F.A., van Driel, M.L., Arroll, B. et al. (2012). Analysis of decisions made in meta-analyses of depression screening and the risk of confirmation bias: a case study. *BMC Med. Res. Methodol.* https://doi.org/10.1186/1471-2288-12-76.

161. Shepperd, J.A., Waters, E.A., Weinstein, N.D. et al. (2015). A primer on unrealistic optimism. *Curr. Dir. Psychol. Sci.* 24: 232–237.

162. Sharot, T. (2011). The optimism bias. *Curr. Biol.* 21: R941–R945.

163. Zakeri, K., Noticewala, S.S., Vitzthum, L.K. et al. (2018). 'Optimism bias' in contemporary national clinical trial network phase III trials: are we improving? *Ann. Oncol.* 29: 2135–2139.

164. Djulbegovic, B., Kumar, A., Magazin, A. et al. (2011). Optimism bias leads to inconclusive results-an empirical study. *J. Clin. Epidemiol.* 64: 583–593.

165. Knottnerus, J.A. and Tugwell, P. (2016). Prevention of premature trial discontinuation: how to counter Lasagna's law. *J. Clin. Epidemiol.* 80: 1–2.

166. Blank, H., Musch, J., and Pohl, R.F. (2007). Hindsight bias: on being wise after the event. *Soc. Cogn.* 25: 1–9.

167. Roese, N.J. and Vohs, K.D. (2012). Hindsight bias. *Perspect. Psychol. Sci.* 7: 411–426.

168. Effron, D.A. and Conway, P. (2015). When virtue leads to villainy: advances in research on moral self-licensing. *Curr. Opin. Psychol.* 6: 32–35.

169. Blanken, I., van de Ven, N., and Zeelenberg, M. (2015). A meta-analytic review of moral licensing. *Personal. Soc. Psychol. Bull.* 41: 540–558.

170. Gunsalus, C.K. and Robinson, A.D. (2018). Nine pitfalls of research misconduct. *Nature* 557: 297–299.

171. Franzen, M., Rodder, S., and Weingart, P. (2007). Fraud: causes and culprits as perceived by science and the media. Institutional changes, rather than individual motivations, encourage misconduct. *EMBO Rep.* 8: 3–7.

172. Bouter, L.M. (2015). Commentary: perverse incentives or rotten apples? *Account Res.* 22: 148–161.

173. Yarborough, M., Nadon, R., and Karlin, D.G. (2019). Four erroneous beliefs thwarting more trustworthy research. *elife* https://doi.org/10.7554/eLife.45261.

174. Holtfreter, K., Reisig, M.D., Pratt, T.C. et al. (2019). The perceived causes of research misconduct among faculty members in the natural, social, and applied sciences. *Stud. High. Educ.* https://doi.org/10.1080/03075079.2019.1593352.

CHAPTER 8

Developing a Strategy to Prevent Poor Quality and Misleading Research

A major aim of this book was to evaluate the statement made by Roberts and colleagues, that 'the knowledge system underpinning healthcare is not fit for purpose and must change' [1]. The conclusion is an unqualified yes, the evidence base for treatments has many serious deficiencies. The findings presented in this book highlight the need for radical change to improve the quality of medical research. The previous chapters have explored the nature and causes of waste and distortion, providing a starting point for action. (For ease of reference, the main findings about poor quality research, and its causes, are summarised in Appendix 1.)

There are no simple ways of preventing the many flaws that threaten the validity of medical research. To date, many initiatives have been proposed to tackle poor quality and misleading research. Appendix 2 provides an extensive list of these. The examination of

Evidence in Medicine: The Common Flaws, Why They Occur and How to Prevent Them, First Edition. Iain K Crombie.
© 2021 John Wiley & Sons Ltd. Published 2021 by John Wiley & Sons Ltd.

the causes of the deficiencies in medical evidence (in previous chapters) has confirmed that actions are needed in three major areas: the research environment; research oversight and research integrity. The proposed initiatives in Appendix 2 identify a fourth topic, research transparency. Together, these are the areas in which decisive action is needed to improve the quality of evidence in medicine. Thus, the initiatives in Appendix 2 have been organised in the four categories: the research environment; research transparency; research oversight and research integrity.

The diversity of factors that contribute to wasted and misleading research confirm the need for an overarching strategy of coherent, synergistic actions. This chapter outlines the way such a strategy could be developed. It briefly describes the four major categories for action, and reviews initiatives from each group. This highlights the challenges to implementing change, which in turn identifies the essential elements of a strategy to transform medical research. The chapter concludes with an agenda for action.

RESEARCH ENVIRONMENT

The research environment is highly competitive, in which researchers are under considerable pressure to gain grants, conduct studies and publish results. This creates the incentive to manipulate the research process to ensure that the criteria for success in applications for jobs, promotion and tenure are met. To highlight some key challenges for implementation, two initiatives are reviewed for this category: research assessment and research training.

Research Assessment

Researchers are assessed by the number of papers published, and whether these are in prestigious journals and are subsequently highly cited [2]. This focus on publication metrics is widely recognised to encourage research behaviours that furnish impressive findings rather than rigorous studies [3, 4]. The Declaration of Research Assessment (DORA) in 2012 [5] and subsequent statements such as the Hong Kong Principles [6] make a clear commitment to replacing publication metrics with measures that assess the rigour and value of research. These statements are not always translated into action: a recent survey of academic institutions showed that the traditional measures (e.g. publications, authorship order, journal impact factor, grant funding) were commonly used [7]. In contrast non-traditional measures (e.g. registering research, adhering to reporting guidelines or data sharing) were seldom mentioned.

What is lacking are mechanisms for implementing the DORA and Hong Kong principles, together with methods of auditing subsequent changes. It will be a formidable task to persuade all research institutions, and their appointments committees, to modify their methods of assessment. The medical journals and funding bodies would also need to give enthusiastic support to this initiative. In effect there needs to be a wholesale change in the research culture. Without enthusiastic support, the DORA Declaration could remain a laudable goal, rather than a transformative principle.

Research Training

Many of the weaknesses in medical evidence can be linked to inadequate knowledge and understanding of the research process. For example, the common problem of failing to recruit the intended number of participants to a trial suggests limited knowledge of the literature on effective interventions to increase recruitment, and a lack of awareness of the importance of careful piloting of study methods. Similarly inadequate descriptions of randomisation and blinding procedures may reflect unfamiliarity with trial reporting procedures. Training for researchers is frequently proposed as a way of improving the design and conduct of research [8–13].

Researcher training could cover the design features of the main study methods (trials, systematic reviews, cohort, case control and surveys), and their common pitfalls. In addition, training could cover the fundamental principles of rigorous research, as well as the proper interpretation of uncertainty and the motivation to identify inconsistencies in findings [14]. Given the frequency with which unhelpful or poor quality studies are published, this training is urgently needed.

The process of developing and delivering training raises several challenges: how will researchers who need training be identified and motivated to engage in educational activities; who will develop the teaching materials and how would they be delivered; what should be the balance between didactic and experiential learning; should mentors be involved in the training and, if so, how would they be identified; who would administer the process; and how would the impact of the training be audited. These are difficult questions, but the answers will certainly involve: availability of individuals skilled in research training; methods to ensure compliance of researchers, either by incentivising or mandatory measures; willingness of experienced researchers to act as mentors; and substantial financial support. The institutions that carry out the research are clearly in the best position to coordinate the development and delivery of this training [14, 15], but they will need additional funds to deliver effective training.

RESEARCH TRANSPARENCY

To enable the quality of research to be assessed, the study design, the methods used, the data collected, the analyses conducted and the logic of interpretation should be available to other researchers. This is research transparency. Three initiatives, trial registration, trial reporting and data sharing, are explored to identify some of barriers, and potential solutions, to increased transparency.

Trial Registration

Before beginning a clinical trial, researchers are strongly encouraged to record the study methods in one of the international trial registries [16]. Registration ensures that key features of the design are specified before any participants are recruited to the study. Comparing the final report with the registered information identifies deviations from the original plan, such as outcome switching or changes to the statistical analysis plan. Registration would also provide searchable databases of all trials for those conducting systematic reviews of specific treatments. In practice, the frequency of trial registration is low. One study found that although about ½ of trials are registered, only 20% do so prospectively [17]; a more recent study found that 42% were prospectively registered [18]. Even when registration is made a condition for ethical approval, some 20% of trials are still not registered [19].

Researchers give several reasons for failing to comply with registration requirements: lack of awareness, a simple omission, difficulties with the process and lack of time [18, 20]. These explanations are not what would be expected from competent researchers keen to attain the highest standards of trial conduct. Possibly the pressures of their competitive environment encourage a focus on completing and publishing trials, with less attention given to procedural issues such as registration. This would explain why repeated exhortations to adhere to guidelines are often ignored. Some form of sanction could be used for those who do not comply [19]; one option would be to make registration a legal requirement with fines for those who do not comply. Another approach would be to emphasise the importance of trial registration in the training of researchers.

Quality of Reporting of Trial Methods

The improvement in the reporting of trial methodology is one of the major successes of the quest for high quality research. Since the advent of the CONSORT statement, which clearly describes how each element of the study design should be presented, substantial improvements have occurred. But, many trial reports still contain unclear methodology, most notably for those items associated with increased risk of bias [21]. In addition, the reporting of harms and of the description of statistical methods is frequently suboptimal [22, 23]. Possible explanations for these shortcomings include that authors are unaware of, or choose to ignore, reporting guidelines, and that journal editors and their peer reviewers do not enforce them. These findings indicate the need for further training of researchers, and for methods to encourage or enforce compliance with the accepted standards for reporting.

Data Sharing

Sharing of the data from a study with other researchers is seen as essential to research transparency [24]. Reanalysis allows others to check the results from the original report. Many national and international agencies have supported the sharing of data from clinical trials [25–27], and substantial progress has been made to identify appropriate principles and safeguards [28–30].

Currently the rates of data sharing are low [31]. Researchers are reluctant to share their data because of lack of time and the absence of training and facilities to support the process. In addition, the potential for negative consequences of data sharing and the lack of benefit for doing so are major barriers to data sharing [32, 33]. Data sharing also requires the cooperation of many stakeholders, the provision of computing and data handling expertise, and funding for infrastructure and staff costs. Until these issues are resolved, rates of sharing are likely to remain low.

RESEARCH OVERSIGHT

The experience of the financial sector is that misconduct is common when supervision is lax. The evidence on questionable research practices, data manipulation and data fraud clearly shows that these unacceptable behaviours are common in research. The hypercompetitive research environment and an oversight system based on trust provide the incentive and the opportunity for misconduct. New methods need to be implemented to detect lapses from conventional standards, so that the likelihood of being found out acts as a powerful deterrent. A host of initiatives have been launched to improve research oversight (see Appendix 2), of which two initiatives are reviewed: peer review and selective outcome reporting.

Strengthen Peer Review

Peer review is used by journals to ensure the value of the papers they publish [34], although there is little evidence that it improves the quality of published studies [35]. Many editors think that peer review should assess the importance, novelty and relevance of the study to their journal rather than checking adherence to reporting guidelines [36]. Further, evaluating the risk of bias and checking the adequacy of outcome reporting are often given a low priority by editors [37].

Several initiatives have been proposed to strengthen peer review, including general training of the reviewers [38], and creating new specialist reviewers who would focus on particular study designs [39]. Another approach is to involve trial methodologists or statisticians in the review process [40]. The use of web-based support tools has also shown promise for improving adherence to reporting guidelines [41, 42].

These new ideas could change the nature of peer review from a system based on trust [43], to a 'trust, but verify model' [44]. The process will require a major revision to the roles of editors and reviewers, and will incur training and running costs. At present journals find it difficult to recruit reviewers [45], and the additional workload of verification will exacerbate this. A possible solution would be to provide sufficient professional reward to compensate reviewers for their time. Improving peer review will also need a substantial number of trial methodologists and statisticians, who may have to be paid for their efforts. Strengthened peer review will involve cost and behaviour change.

Monitor Selective Outcome Reporting

In clinical trials, the outcome measures identified at the design stage are frequently changed by the time the study is published. One way to prevent this would be to monitor trials, at the time of submission of manuscripts to journals, asking authors to explain any changes identified [46]. With over 20,000 trials published each year [47], the task of assessing them would be a labour of Hercules. The process would also require the support of all medical journals, which would have to accept the administrative inconvenience, and the inevitable delay in publishing manuscripts. In addition, teams of researchers with appropriate expertise would be needed to carry out the work.

RESEARCH INTEGRITY

Concerns about data fabrication and falsification led to the creation of the Office of Research Integrity in the USA [48], and many other countries now have policies on research integrity [49–53]. Since 2007, the World Conferences on Research Integrity have debated and promoted integrity policies [54]. These are important developments but further actions are needed. To illustrate the challenges to improving research integrity, two groups of initiatives are reviewed: those aimed at reducing spin and those to improve the reporting of conflict of interest.

Reduce the Use of Spin

Spin, exaggeration of the value of research, is a common feature of published studies [55, 56]. Researchers may use spin to increase the likelihood of publication in a prestigious journal, and the highly competitive research environment may encourage them to do so. Academic institutions may tolerate spin because it increases the profile of their institutions [57].

Reducing the prevalence of spin will involve ensuring researchers refrain from it when they write papers, and increasing the diligence of journal editors and peer reviewers when they assess manuscripts [56]. It will also need changes to the research environment by removing the incentives for exaggerated conclusions. In short, tackling spin will require a coordinated programme of initiatives designed to change the behaviour of several professional groups. This is a formidable task, which will require careful negotiation with key stakeholders and combination of incentives and sanctions to encourage compliance.

Reporting Conflict of Interest

Financial conflicts of interest (CoIs) are common among authors of research studies, and are often not fully disclosed [58, 59]. Part of the problem is that, although medical journals have policies on reporting conflict of interest [60], it is unclear whether they verify authors' statements. Further, few journals require authors to describe the nature of their conflict of interest [61]. There is compelling evidence that financial CoIs, whether reported or not, increase the likelihood of drawing positive conclusions [62, 63]. The finding that systematic reviews almost always ignore the financial CoIs reported in the primary papers [64–66], suggests that the evidence base may be biased.

Currently, disclosure of CoIs 'does not reduce or eliminate bias' [67]. To overcome this problem, one suggestion is to disregard all research with CoIs [67]. This is not an ideal approach; although it would eliminate biased studies, it could also exclude many unbiased trials and systematic reviews. Another approach would be to make disclosures more meaningful, by explaining the context of the CoI [68]. Each author could describe their role in the research, and how the CoI might have influenced the conduct of the study or interpretation of the findings. This would increase the visibility to readers, and possibly alter their interpretation of the findings. The impact of this approach would need to be tested before being adopted. Its implementation would also need the support of journal editors and researchers. At present, conflict of interest is an unsolved problem.

Integrity Training

Many training programmes have been developed to improve research integrity, but these vary greatly in in content, delivery methods and quality [69, 70]. There is little evidence that integrity training is effective [71], and some evidence that it can be counterproductive [72]. Further, researchers often have little confidence in the ability of training to improve research integrity [73]. New approaches are needed. Integrity issues could be incorporated into a broader training in research, rather than reducing its relevance to researchers by treating it as a separate topic. More importantly, the mismatch between the causes of misconduct (the competitive research environment) and the nature of the training (education on the importance of integrity) needs to be addressed [74]. Researchers are likely to disregard approaches that place responsibility solely on individuals, rather than addressing problems in the system in which they function [75]. As with all new training, extra resource will be needed for development and delivery and the evaluation of its outcomes.

ESSENTIAL ELEMENTS OF A TRANSFORMATIONAL STRATEGY

Many excellent suggestions have been made to improve research quality: what is lacking are the methods to implement them. The preceding brief review of initiatives highlights many challenges to the implementation of initiatives to transform unhelpful and misleading research. To be successful, six key issues need to be addressed: commitment from key stakeholders, monitoring the research process, sanctions and incentives, availability of expertise, coordinated approaches and financial support.

Commitment from Key Stakeholders

A key requirement for action is enthusiastic commitment from the key stakeholders. These comprise all the groups involved in the research process: funding agencies, medical publishers, regulatory agencies, and the researchers and their institutions [76–79]. The motives, concerns and aspirations of individual stakeholders need to be fully understood to ensure their commitment. It is easy to propose that particular agencies, such as medical journals, funding bodies or research ethics committees, should be involved in delivering initiatives. These organisations might seem ideally placed for this work, because they have direct involvement in the research process. However these groups already fill important roles, which come with pressures and deadlines. It is unrealistic to expect them to shoulder a substantial additional burden: they would need to be persuaded of the benefits of taking action, and provided with sufficient support to ensure their existing priorities will not be affected.

One issue on which it may be difficult to gain commitment is the seductive allure of novel, exciting findings. Everybody wants to be associated with apparently groundbreaking studies: researchers know they are the key to a successful career; funding agencies and research institutions benefit from increased prestige, and medical journals gain both prestige and financial success. By comparison, a focus on more the mundane but more important issue, rigour of the research methods, will have little appeal. The tension between exciting findings and methodological rigour is possibly the most important problem that the key stakeholders need to resolve.

Monitoring the Research Process

The process of ensuring the trustworthiness of research will require systematically checking trial registration and publication, comparing proposed methods with what was actually done and searching for flaws and inconsistencies in study reports. This is likely to be unpopular among key stakeholders. Researchers may dislike the implied lack of trust inherent in auditing the conduct of their studies; they may also complain about the imposition of another administrative hurdle to be overcome. Research organisations could have similar concerns, but may also regard auditing as a lowly form of academic bookkeeping. It will appear remote from their mission statements, which focus on advancing knowledge and contributing to human well-being. Given the parlous state of medical evidence, routine auditing may be the only way to ensure, and to demonstrate, that research can be trusted. Persuading the key stakeholders of the need for it will be challenging.

Sanctions and Incentives

Evaluations of important initiatives, such as adherence to CONSORT, registering and timely publication of trials, and data sharing, consistently conclude that their implementation could be improved. Sanctions are often suggested to increase adherence to these reforms. In the US financial sanctions for the reporting of trial results have been incorporated into law. However these were not enforced and reporting rates remained poor. As DeVito and colleagues concluded for trial reporting, 'trial reporting will only improve when regulators routinely impose fines and other sanctions' [80]. This is likely to be true of other recommended actions such as registering of protocol and statistical analysis plans.

Sanctions need not be financial. Researchers and research institutions value their reputations. The threat of being placed on a publicly available blacklist for behaviours, such as failing to publish trial results in a timely manner, could incentivise change. Similarly, medical journals could be held to account for tardy publication of corrections to errors, or retractions of flawed papers. The key requirements for effective sanctions are that they target issues that are important to stakeholders and that they are vigorously implemented. They should also be sensitively negotiated.

Availability of Expertise

Many initiatives call for closer scrutiny of the research process. This will require individuals with expertise in clinical trials, systematic reviews, statistical analysis, reporting guidelines and software engineering. It may be unreasonable to expect existing experts to undertake such tasks; given the pressures in the research environment, those with relevant expertise may be unwilling to sacrifice their research time. Some form of valued professional recognition could encourage engagement in this work.

Other initiatives require educationalists to deliver effective training on topics including study design, reporting guidelines and research integrity. In addition, implementing many initiatives will require skilled negotiators to engender commitment among key stakeholders. In short, large numbers of highly skilled individuals will needed to deliver the improvement agenda. It is unrealistic to expect them to take on onerous tasks in addition to their existing workload. Recruitment and training of new staff may be the only solution.

Coordinated Approaches

Improving research quality with several individual initiatives would be far less effective than a well-planned coordinated approach. For example, on their own, training courses to improve research integrity will have limited effect, but would act synergistically with other initiatives such as monitoring data quality, promoting the reporting of misconduct and certification of research integrity by a senior member of the research institution. In addition, efforts to promote integrity would be more effective if the perverse incentives were removed. Organising the implementation of groups of initiatives will require concerted action at a senior level.

Incentives for desired behaviours could also be used synergistically with sanctions for poor behaviour. For example, incentives could be offered for actions such as pre-registering a study, publishing a null result or making study data publically available in the criteria for staff recruitment and promotion. Simultaneously making the failure to take these actions a threat to the reputation of individuals and institutions could increase willingness to implement change. Researchers have responded enthusiastically to the perverse incentives of impact factors by gaming the citation process; they are likely to respond to a revised incentive structure.

Combining initiatives can also be more economical. For example, the monitoring of outcome switching and of adherence to a pre-specified statistical analysis plan both require searching trial registries and looking for published protocols. These activities could easily be combined with checking registration status of the trial and adherence to the CONSORT statement, as all these activities involve searching for supporting documents and careful reading of the final study report. Establishing small teams with appropriate expertise would facilitate a single pass approach to implement several initiatives.

Financial Support

The effective delivery of many initiatives will require substantial financial support, raising the question of where will the money come from? Before answering that question, it is worth considering the cost of not taking action.

The Cost of Inaction

At present many billions of dollars are spent on medical research. The global expenditure on biomedical research was estimated at $268.4 billion in 2012 [81], since when it is likely to have increased. For example the US National Institutes of Health has an annual budget of over $37 billion for 2019 [82], and in the UK two organisations, the MRC and NIHR, have a joint spend of almost $2 billion [83, 84] and the medical charities contribute over $3 billion (www.amrc.org.uk/pages/category/member-directory?Take=20). The pharmaceutical industry spends substantially more than governments, amounting to over $150 billion in 2016 [85].

One group estimated that 85% of research was wasted [8], so it is possible that a similar proportion of research spend is wasted. Based on that estimate, some $228.1 billion of the $268.4 in 2012 was wasted. Even if the extent of waste was more modest, say, 20%, this would still amount to about $53.7 billion of waste. The question then becomes how much are we prepared to spend to prevent waste. Would an annual investment of $1 billion be worthwhile if it prevented $5 billion of wasted research? This simple calculation illustrates an important point: major investment in research quality would be worthwhile, even if it had only a modest impact on wasted and misleading research.

Who Should Pay?

The question of who should pay can be answered by considering who currently pays for, and who profits from, research. In many countries, governments provide direct support to universities as well as supporting research through sponsored funding bodies. These efforts benefit the economy and improve the health and well-being of the public. The pharmaceutical and medical devices industries invest heavily in research, with the aim of profiting from interventions that improve the quality of life and save lives. Similarly, many charitable organisations provide funding for research into effective treatments, with the aim of benefiting patients. Finally there is the publishing industry: a lucrative business field with profit margins as high as 40% [86]. Asking for a contribution from publishers towards improving research quality does not seem unreasonable. As all these organisations benefit from research, it would be in their interests to contribute to cost-effective methods of increasing the amount of high quality research. The maxim, each according to their means, would be appropriate here.

A possible mechanism for funding would be to top slice a small proportion of the budgets of funding bodies, diverting the money to research improvement activities. This would reduce the direct spending on research, but would be more than compensated for by the increase in the number of high quality studies. Rather than specifying arbitrary proportions, the sums involved would be determined by the cost of programmes of initiatives. The setting up costs of some programmes could be high, but these would fall as they become embedded in the research process. Recognising this, a phased approach with groups of initiatives implemented sequentially, would avoid unreasonably high initial costs.

IMPLEMENTING A PROGRAMME FOR ACTION

This chapter has outlined a framework to create the 'innovative, collaborative and coordinated approaches .... that boost the quality, relevance and reliability of all research' [87]. The main barrier to improving research quality is not a lack of ideas, Appendix 2 describes a wealth of initiatives; the difficulty lies in the implementing these proposals. Many of the shortcomings in research are messy problems: they are multifaceted, with limited evidence about their causes and involve multiple stakeholders who have conflicting goals. Although improving the quality of research is in the interests of all the stakeholders, there is likely to be considerable resistance to changing current practices. Solving these problems requires negotiation, judgement, combinations of initiatives and funding.

Together the key stakeholders could forge strategies to improve the quality of research. The implementation of most of the initiatives to improve research quality will require changes in the values, beliefs and attitudes of these stakeholders. The process could begin by valuing the important contributions that all these groups have made to the many successes of medical research. It could then review how wasted and poor quality impedes attainment of their mission statements. Contributing to improvement programmes then becomes an opportunity for the stakeholders to increase the value of their work.

The process of change could be organised in stages. Leaders from each stakeholder group could meet to discuss general principles and negotiate agreement on the need for action. In turn, working groups could identify implementation programmes, which would be negotiated with the stakeholder groups. The result would be an overarching strategy supported by detailed proposals. In overview, the sequence of actions would be:

- create a coherent and comprehensive programme of detailed proposals to tackle the causes of poor quality research
- ensure that appropriate incentives and sanctions are identified
- review the resources and the expertise required for each programme
- prioritise initiatives, and groups of initiatives, by feasibility (resources required, ease of implementation) and likely impact
- canvas support from the stakeholders, modifying proposals to accommodate their needs
- specify a timetable with development and implementation phases
- evaluate the impact of each group of initiatives, modifying them in the light of the findings

The present crisis in evidence requires decisive action. The programme for change will be expensive, albeit the sums involved will be small in comparison with the total research spend, and the cost of wasted research. Only with the wholehearted commitment of all the stakeholders will we achieve high quality evidence for healthcare. Medical research has a duty to consistently provide reliable results, and at present it is failing to do so: patients and the general population deserve better.

REFERENCES

1. Roberts, I., Ker, K., Edwards, P. et al. (2015). The knowledge system underpinning healthcare is not fit for purpose and must change. *BMJ* https://doi.org/10.1136/bmj.h2463.

2. Moher, D., Naudet, F., Cristea, I.A. et al. (2018). Assessing scientists for hiring, promotion, and tenure. *PLoS Biol.* https://doi.org/10.1371/journal.pbio.2004089.

3. Lindner, M.D., Torralba, K.D., and Khan, N.A. (2018). Scientific productivity: an exploratory study of metrics and incentives. *PLoS One* https://doi.org/10.1371/journal.pone.0195321.

4. Higginson, A.D. and Munafo, M.R. (2016). Current incentives for scientists lead to underpowered studies with erroneous conclusions. *PLoS Biol.* https://doi.org/10.1371/journal.pbio.1002106.

5. Anoymous (2012). *San Francisco Declaration on Research Assessment.* https://sfdora.org. Accessed 19 December 2019.

6. Moher, D., Bouter, L., Kleinert, S. et al. (2020). The Hong Kong principles for assessing researchers: fostering research integrity. *PLoS Biol.* https://doi.org/10.1371/journal.pbio.3000737.

7. Rice, D.B., Raffoul, H., Ioannidis, J.P.A. et al. (2020). Academic criteria for promotion and tenure in biomedical sciences faculties: cross sectional analysis of international sample of universities. *BMJ* https://doi.org/10.1136/bmj.m2081.

8. Chalmers, I. and Glasziou, P. (2009). Avoidable waste in the production and reporting of research evidence. *Lancet* 374: 86–89.

9. Casadevall, A. and Fang, F.C. (2018). Making the scientific literature fail-safe. *J. Clin. Invest.* 128: 4243–4244.

10. Ioannidis, J.P., Fanelli, D., Dunne, D.D. et al. (2015). *PLoS Biol.* https://doi.org/10.1371/journal.pbio.1002264.

11. Glasziou, P., Altman, D.G., Bossuyt, P. et al. (2014). Reducing waste from incomplete or unusable reports of biomedical research. *Lancet* 383: 267–276.

12. Page, M.J. and Moher, D. (2016). Mass production of systematic reviews and meta-analyses: an exercise in mega-silliness? *Milbank Q.* 94: 515–519.

13. Li, G., Bhatt, M., Wang, M. et al. (2018). Enhancing primary reports of randomized controlled trials: three most common challenges and suggested solutions. *Proc. Natl. Acad. Sci. U. S. A.* 115: 2595–2599.

14. Koroshetz, W.J., Behrman, S., Brame, C.J. et al. (2020). Framework for advancing rigorous research. *elife* https://doi.org/10.7554/eLife.55915.

15. Begley, C.G., Buchan, A.M., and Dirnagl, U. (2015). Institutions must do their part for reproducibility. *Nature* 525: 25–27.

16. Pansieri, C., Pandolfini, C., and Bonati, M. (2015). The evolution in registration of clinical trials: a chronicle of the historical calls and current initiatives promoting transparency. *Eur. J. Clin. Pharmacol.* 71: 1159–1164.

17. Trinquart, L., Dunn, A.G., and Bourgeois, F.T. (2018). Registration of published randomized trials: a systematic review and meta-analysis. *BMC Med.* https://doi.org/10.1186/s12916-018-1168-6.

18. Al-Durra, M., Nolan, R.P., Seto, E. et al. (2020). Prospective registration and reporting of trial number in randomised clinical trials: global cross sectional study of the adoption of ICMJE and declaration of Helsinki recommendations. *BMJ* https://doi.org/10.1136/bmj.m982.

19. Denneny, C., Bourne, S., and Kolstoe, S.E. (2019). Registration audit of clinical trials given a favourable opinion by UK research ethics committees. *BMJ Open* https://doi.org/10.1136/bmjopen-2018-026840.

20. Hunter, K.E., Seidler, A.L., and Askie, L.M. (2018). Prospective registration trends, reasons for retrospective registration and mechanisms to increase prospective registration compliance: descriptive analysis and survey. *BMJ Open* https://doi.org/10.1136/bmjopen-2017-019983.

21. Dechartres, A., Trinquart, L., Atal, I. et al. (2017). Evolution of poor reporting and inadequate methods over time in 20 920 randomised controlled trials included in Cochrane reviews: research on research study. *BMJ* https://doi.org/10.1136/bmj.j2490.

22. Golder, S., Loke, Y.K., Wright, K. et al. (2016). Reporting of adverse events in published and unpublished studies of health care interventions: a systematic review. *PLoS Med.* https://doi.org/10.1371/journal.pmed.1002127.

23. Lindsey, M.L., Gray, G.A., Wood, S.K. et al. (2018). Statistical considerations in reporting cardiovascular research. *Am. J. Physiol. Heart Circ. Physiol.* https://doi.org/10.1152/ajpheart.00309.2018.

24. Bauchner, H., Golub, R.M., and Fontanarosa, P.B. (2016). Data sharing: an ethical and scientific imperative. *JAMA* 315: 1237–1239.

25. Lo, B. (2015). Sharing clinical trial data: maximizing benefits, minimizing risk. *JAMA* 313: 793–794.

26. Taichman, D.B., Sahni, P., Pinborg, A. et al. (2017). Data sharing statements for clinical trials. *BMJ* https://doi.org/10.1136/bmj.c117.

27. Yancy, C.W., Harrington, R.A., and Bonow, R.O. (2018). Data sharing-the time has (not yet?) come. *JAMA Cardiol.* 3: 797–798.

28. Boeckhout, M., Zielhuis, G.A., and Bredenoord, A.L. (2018). The FAIR guiding principles for data stewardship: fair enough? *Eur. J. Hum. Genet.* 26: 931–936.

29. Ohmann, C., Banzi, R., Canham, S. et al. (2107). Sharing and reuse of individual participant data from clinical trials: principles and recommendations. *BMJ Open* https://doi.org/10.1136/bmjopen-2017-018647.

30. Ross, J.S., Waldstreicher, J., Bamford, S. et al. (2018). Overview and experience of the YODA project with clinical trial data sharing after 5 years. *Sci. Data* https://doi.org/10.1038/sdata.2018.268.

31. Rowhani-Farid, A., Allen, M., and Barnett, A.G. (2017). What incentives increase data sharing in health and medical research? A systematic review. *Res. Integr. Peer Rev.* https://doi.org/10.1186/s41073-017-0028-9.

32. Chawinga, W.C. and Zinn, S. (2019). Global perspectives of research data sharing: a systematic literature review. *Libr. Inf. Sci. Res.* 41: 109–122.

33. Krahe, M.A., Wolski, M., Mickan, S. et al. (2020). Developing a strategy to improve data sharing in health research: a mixedmethods study to identify barriers and facilitators. *Health Inf. Manage. J.* https://doi.org/10.1177/1833358320917207.

34. Horbach, S. and Halffman, W.W. (2018). The changing forms and expectations of peer review. *Res. Integr. Peer Rev.* https://doi.org/10.1186/s41073-018-0051-5.

35. Bruce, R., Chauvin, A., Trinquart, L. et al. (2016). Impact of interventions to improve the quality of peer review of biomedical journals: a systematic review and meta-analysis. *BMC Med.* https://doi.org/10.1186/s12916-016-0631-5.

36. Blanco, D., Hren, D., Kirkham, J.J. et al. (2019). A survey exploring biomedical editors' perceptions of editorial interventions to

improve adherence to reporting guidelines. *F1000Res.* https://doi.org/10.12688/f1000research.20556.3.

37. Chauvin, A., Ravaud, P., Baron, G. et al. (2015). The most important tasks for peer reviewers evaluating a randomized controlled trial are not congruent with the tasks most often requested by journal editors. *BMC Med.* https://doi.org/10.1186/s12916-015-0395-3.

38. Moher, D. and Altman, D.G. (2015). Four proposals to help improve the medical research literature. *PLoS Med.* https://doi.org/10.1371/journal.pmed.1001864.

39. Patel, J. (2014). Why training and specialization is needed for peer review: a case study of peer review for randomized controlled trials. *BMC Med.* https://doi.org/10.1186/s12916-014-0128-z.

40. Krummel, M., Blish, C., Kuhns, M. et al. (2019). Universal principled review: a community-driven method to improve peer review. *Cell* 179: 1441–1445.

41. Blanco, D., Schroter, S., Aldcroft, A. et al. (2020). Effect of an editorial intervention to improve the completeness of reporting of randomised trials: a randomised controlled trial. *BMJ Open* https://doi.org/10.1136/bmjopen-2020-036799.

42. Hopewell, S., Boutron, I., Altman, D. et al. (2016). Impact of a web-based tool (WebCONSORT) to improve the reporting of randomised trials: results of a randomised controlled trial. *BMC Med.* https://doi.org/10.1186/s12916-016-0736-x.

43. Hames, I. (2014). Peer review at the beginning of the 21st century. *Sci. Ed.* 1: 4–8.

44. Lee, C.J. and Moher, D. (2017). Promote scientific integrity through journal peer review data. *Science* 357: 256–257.

45. Malcom, D. (2018). It's time we fix the peer review system. *Am. J. Pharm. Educ.* 82: 385–387.

46. Ioannidis, J.P., Caplan, A.L., and Dal-Re, R. (2017). Outcome reporting bias in clinical trials: why monitoring matters. *BMJ* https://doi.org/10.1136/bmj.j408.

47. Niforatos, J.D., Weaver, M., and Johansen, M.E. (2019). Assessment of publication trends of systematic reviews and randomized clinical trials, 1995 to 2017. *JAMA Intern. Med.* 179: 1593–1594.

48. Price, A.R. (2013). Research misconduct and its federal regulation: the origin and history of the Office of Research Integrity – with personal views by ORI's former associate director for investigative oversight. *Account Res.* 20: 291–319.

49. Khajuria, A. and Agha, R. (2014). Fraud in scientific research – birth of the concordat to uphold research integrity in the United Kingdom. *J. R. Soc. Med.* 107: 61–65.

50. Tavare, A. (2011). Managing research misconduct: is anyone getting it right? *BMJ* https://doi.org/10.1136/bmj.d8212.

51. Godecharle, S., Nemery, B., and Dierickx, K. (2013). Guidance on research integrity: no union in Europe. *Lancet* 381: 1097–1098.

52. Torjesen, I. (2012). Strategy for boosting integrity of research is launched in UK. *BMJ* https://doi.org/10.1136/bmj.e4747.

53. Bonn, N.A., Godecharle, S., and Dierickx, K. (2017). European Universities' guidance on research integrity and misconduct: accessibility, approaches, and content. *J. Empir. Res. Hum. Res. Ethics* 12: 33–44.

54. Anderson, M.S. (2014). Global research integrity in relation to the United States' research-integrity infrastructure. *Account Res.* 21: 1–8.

55. Millar, N., Salager-Meyer, F., and Budgell, B. (2019). "It is important to reinforce the importance of …": 'hype' in reports of randomized controlled trials. *Engl. Specif. Purp.* 54: 139–151.

56. Boutron, I. and Ravaud, P. (2018). Misrepresentation and distortion of research in biomedical literature. *Proc. Natl. Acad. Sci. U. S. A.* 115: 2613–2619.

57. Hopf, H., Matlin, S.A., Mehta, G. et al. (2020). Blocking the hype-hypocrisy-falsification-fakery pathway is needed to safeguard science. *Angew. Chem. Int. Ed.* 59: 2150–2154.

58. Bauchner, H., Fontanarosa, P.B., and Flanagin, A. (2018). Conflicts of interests, authors, and journals new challenges for a persistent problem. *JAMA* 320: 2315–2318.

59. Cherla, D.V., Olavarria, O.A., Holihan, J.L. et al. (2017). Discordance of conflict of interest self-disclosure and the centers of Medicare and Medicaid services. *J. Surg. Res.* 218: 18–22.

60. Shawwa, K., Kallas, R., Koujanian, S. et al. (2016). Requirements of clinical journals for Authors' disclosure of financial and

non-financial conflicts of interest: a cross sectional study. *PLoS One* https://doi.org/10.1371/journal.pone.0152301.

61. Khamis, A.M., Hakoum, M.B., Bou-Karroum, L. et al. (2017). Requirements of health policy and services journals for authors to disclose financial and non-financial conflicts of interest: a cross-sectional study. *Health Res. Policy Syst.* https://doi.org/10.1186/s12961-017-0244-2.

62. Cherla, D.V., Viso, C.P., Olavarria, O.A. et al. (2018). The impact of financial conflict of interest on surgical research: an observational study of published manuscripts. *World J. Surg.* 42: 2757–2762.

63. Cherla, D.V., Viso, C.P., Holihan, J.L. et al. (2019). The effect of financial conflict of interest, disclosure status, and relevance on medical research from the United States. *J. Gen. Intern. Med.* 34: 429–434.

64. Elia, N., von Elm, E., Chatagner, A. et al. (2016). How do authors of systematic reviews deal with research malpractice and misconduct in original studies? A cross-sectional analysis of systematic reviews and survey of their authors. *BMJ Open* https://doi.org/10.1136/bmjopen-2015-010442.

65. Faggion, C.M. Jr., Monje, A., and Wasiak, J. (2018). Appraisal of systematic reviews on the management of peri-implant diseases with two methodological tools. *J. Clin. Periodontol.* 45: 754–766.

66. Benea, C., Turner, K.A., Roseman, M. et al. (2020). Reporting of financial conflicts of interest in meta-analyses of drug trials published in high-impact medical journals: comparison of results from 2017 to 2018 and 2009. *Syst. Rev.* https://doi.org/10.1186/s13643-020-01318-5.

67. Bero, L. (2017). Addressing bias and conflict of interest among biomedical researchers. *JAMA* 317: 1732–1734.

68. Schroter, S., Pakpoor, J., Morris, J. et al. (2019). Effect of different financial competing interest statements on readers' perceptions of clinical educational articles: a randomised controlled trial. *BMJ Open* https://doi.org/10.1136/bmjopen-2018-025029.

69. Steneck, N.H. (2013). Research ethics. Global research integrity training. *Science* 340: 552–553.

70. Kalichman, M. (2014). Rescuing responsible conduct of research (RCR) education. *Account Res.* 21: 68–83.

71. Marusic, A., Wager, E., Utrobicic, A. et al. (2016). Interventions to prevent misconduct and promote integrity in research and publication. *Cochrane Database Syst. Rev.* http://doi.org/10.1002/14651858. MR000038.pub2.

72. Bruton, S.V., Brown, M., Sacco, D.F. et al. (2019). Testing an active intervention to deter researchers' use of questionable research practices. *Res. Integr. Peer Rev.* https://doi.org/10.1186/s41073-019-0085-3.

73. Bruton, S.V., Medlin, M., Brown, M. et al. (2020). Personal motivations and systemic incentives: scientists on questionable research practices. *Sci. Eng. Ethics* 26: 1531–1547.

74. Bonn, N.A. and Pinxten, W. (2019). A decade of empirical research on research integrity: what have we (not) looked at? *J. Empir. Res. Hum. Res. Ethics* 144: 338–352.

75. Davies, S.R. (2019). An ethics of the system: talking to scientists about research integrity. *Sci. Eng. Ethics* 25: 1235–1253.

76. Moher, D., Glasziou, P., Chalmers, I. et al. (2016). Increasing value and reducing waste in biomedical research: who's listening? *Lancet* 387: 1573–1586.

77. Munafo, M.R., Nosek, B.A., Bishop, D.V.M. et al. (2017). A manifesto for reproducible science. *Nat. Hum. Behav.* https://doi.org/10.1038/s41562-016-0021.

78. Bouter, L.M. (2018). Fostering responsible research practices is a shared responsibility of multiple stakeholders. *J. Clin. Epidemiol.* 96: 143–146.

79. Meerpohl, J.J., Schell, L.K., Bassler, D. et al. (2015). Evidence-informed recommendations to reduce dissemination bias in clinical research: conclusions from the OPEN (overcome failure to publish nEgative fiNdings) project based on an international consensus meeting. *BMJ Open* https://doi.org/10.1136/bmjopen-2014-006666.

80. DeVito, N.J., Bacon, S., and Goldacre, B. (2020). Compliance with legal requirement to report clinical trial results on ClinicalTrials. gov: a cohort study. *Lancet* 395: 361–369.

81. Chakma, J., Sun, G.H., Steinberg, J.D. et al. (2014). Asia's ascent – global trends in biomedical R&D expenditures. *N. Engl. J. Med.* 370: 3–6.

82. NIH (2019). *Budget.* https://www.nih.gov/about-nih/what-we-do/budget. Accessed 13 June 2019.

83. Medical Research Council (2018). *Annual report and accounts 2017/18.* London.

84. NIHR (2019). *NIHR Annual Report 2017/18.* www.nihr.ac.uk/about-us/documents/NIHR-Annual-Report-2017-18.pdf. Accessed 13 June 2019.

85. ABPI (2020). *Worlwide pharmaceutical R&D expenditure.* www.abpi.org.uk/facts-and-figures/science-and-innovation/worldwide-pharmaceutical-company-rd-expenditure. Accessed 13 April 2020.

86. Walter, P. and Mullins, D. (2019). From symbiont to parasite: the evolution of for-profit science publishing. *MBoC* 30: 2357–2342.

87. Pilay, D. (2019). Research ethics and integrity challenges require innovative approaches. *Promoting Acad. Integrity* 115: 1–3.

Appendix 1: Summary of the Key Findings on Poor Quality Research

This appendix summarises the findings of Chapters 2–7 on the nature and causes of poor quality and wasted research.

PROBLEMS IN THE DESIGN, CONDUCT, ANALYSIS AND REPORTING OF STUDIES

Trials

Many trials are conducted to a high standard, but a substantial number are of poor quality. Biased trials threaten the delivery of effective healthcare. Wasted trials are a major impediment to progress, squandering resources and betraying the trust of study participants. The inadequacies in the design and conduct of trials may be due to a lack of expertise, inadvertent error or motivated manipulation.

1. Many trials are wasted because:
    (a) previous studies have successfully evaluated the treatment
    (b) deficiencies in the study design or conduct make their findings unreliable

Evidence in Medicine: The Common Flaws, Why They Occur and How to Prevent Them,
First Edition. Iain K Crombie.
© 2021 John Wiley & Sons Ltd. Published 2021 by John Wiley & Sons Ltd.

   (c) the outcome measures that are used have little rele-
        vance to clinicians and patients

   (d) studies are not completed, or their findings are
        not published

2. Sequence generation, allocation concealment, blinding, and
   the methods of following up patients are often poorly
   described or inadequate. These deficiencies can lead to exaggerated estimates of treatment benefit.

3. Substitution of the primary outcome, and selective outcome
   reporting, are common. These actions frequently favour
   significant findings.

4. Adverse events occurring among patients in clinical trials are
   poorly reported. This will bias the benefit-to-harm ratio of
   treatment.

5. Only one half of trials record their details on a clinical trials
   registry. Unregistered trials often report larger effect sizes and
   poorer methodological quality than registered ones.

6. Publication bias, in which non-significant findings are less
   likely to be published, could bias the evidence for treatments.

7. The high frequency of exclusion of certain groups of patients
   (older people and those with comorbidities) could mean that
   the treatment benefits seen in trials are not achieved in routine clinical practice.

8. Trials funded by the pharmaceutical industry generally
   favour the drug that the company manufactures.

Statistical Analysis

The analyses presented in published studies cannot always be taken
at face value. The importance given to $p < 0.05$ is the most likely
driver of statistical misbehaviour.

1. Statistical significance ($p < 0.05$) is widely misinterpreted to
   indicate clinically important treatments. It is only one of several factors that should be considered when evaluating the
   findings of clinical trials.

2. Many trials are too small to reliably identify treatment benefits. These studies are at risk of spurious statistical significance, which can lead to treatments being incorrectly described as effective.

3. There is a marked excess of p-values just below the threshold for statistical significance, and a corresponding deficit just above the threshold. Negative (non-significant) findings are disappearing from published studies.

4. Data analysis provides many opportunities for flexibility in the choice of statistical methods and the ways in which these are employed. Common questionable practices are: deleting selected data points, undeclared multiple testing, biased selection of covariates and inappropriate rounding down of p-values. These can be used to produce misleading statistical significance.

5. Statisticians are sometimes pressured to produce significant findings.

6. Prespecified statistical analysis plans could provide protection against misbehaviours, but most trials do not publish them. When they do, deviations from the plans are common, particularly in choice of covariates and subgroup analysis.

Systematic Reviews

Systematic reviews have the potential to provide reliable evidence on the effectiveness of treatments. Deficiencies in their design, conduct and analysis are common and can bias estimates of treatment benefit.

1. Some systematic reviews are unnecessary replications of previous reviews, such that for some treatments there are many more systematics reviews than there are trials.

2. The processes of searching for relevant trials and extracting the trial data are often poorly conducted. In consequence many systematic reviews may have misleading or unhelpful findings.

3. Insufficient attention is paid to the quality of the trials included in the systematic review. Small trials, and those at high risk of bias, can bias the summary estimate of treatment effect.

4. Heterogeneity across the trials is often poorly addressed, so that the methods of pooling trial findings may be inappropriate.

5. Outcome data are often missing from trials, but this is poorly dealt with by systematic reviews. Failure to address missing data increases the risk of bias in estimates of treatment benefit.

6. The adverse events that are reported in trials are often not included in systematic reviews. This under-reporting will bias the benefit to harms ratio of interventions. The effect will be compounded because trials frequently fail to report harms.

7. Many systematic reviews comprise only a few small trials and cannot provide robust estimates of treatment benefit.

8. Before a full systematic review is conducted, researchers may carry out an initial scoping review to pilot methods and gain an estimate of workload. This prior information could bias the design and conduct of the study.

9. Several stages in the conduct of systematic reviews require judgement (selection of trials for inclusion, choice of outcome measures and decisions on analytic approaches). These provide opportunities for flexibility that can lead to bias.

10. Systematic reviews frequently ignore the conflicts of interest of the authors of the trials included in the review.

FREQUENCY OF DATA FABRICATION AND FALSIFICATION

Researchers frequently admit to, or are shown to have, committed research misconduct. The key findings are:

1. Data fabrication is rare, but can cause serious bias. The true frequency of fabrication will be underestimated because of the difficulty of detecting misbehaviour.

2. Falsification of data and questionable research practices are common and could seriously harm research evidence. Researchers may under-report these behaviours, so that estimates of their frequency could be too low.

3. Data massage, manipulated analyses and selective reporting are easy to do and are unlikely to be detected. These activities distort evidence on effectiveness.

4. Present efforts to detect misconduct are inadequate to the task.

    (a) Researchers are often reluctant to report research misconduct. Most are unaware of the method for reporting it, and systems to support whistleblowers are poor or non-existent.

    (b) Statistical methods to detect data fabrication and falsification are not routinely used.

    (c) Research institutions do not always conduct high quality, full-scale investigations of potential misconduct.

5. Spin, embellishing and exaggerating findings, is common and can mislead. The terms novel, excellent, prominent and unprecedented are frequently used. Non-significant findings are particularly vulnerable to spin.

6. Published studies involving misconduct should be retracted, but this does not always happen. Retracted papers continue to be cited after the misconduct has been reported.

THE CAUSES OF POOR QUALITY AND MISLEADING RESEARCH

The problems of poor quality research are exacerbated by research misconduct, in which the methods, results and reporting of studies are manipulated. The culture of research, and its methods of governance, may foster research misconduct. The characteristics of individuals may also play a role. The key findings are:

1. Large-scale data fabrication is likely to be due to personality disorder, particularly the dark triad of narcissism, Machiavellianism and psychopathy.

2. Small-scale data falsification and questionable research practices are common and may be an accepted, if undesirable, behaviour among many researchers.

3. Novel, exciting, statistically significant findings are the key to career success, including finding a job, being promoted, gaining research grants and being lauded by peers. This provides the incentive for researchers to manipulate data, its analysis and interpretation.

4. The system of research oversight, peer review, is based on trust, and its methods are not designed to detect research malpractice.

5. The researcher has many opportunities for flexibility in the design, conduct and analysis of trials and systematic reviews. Alterations can be easily made to studies, with little chance of being detected.

6. Four factors incentivise questionable research practices and spin.

    (a) the hypercompetitive research environment

    (b) the high value placed on research that is considered excellent

    (c) the use of citation metrics to evaluate research quality

    (d) the low value given to methodologically rigorous studies with negative findings

7. Some researchers choose not to write up negative findings because they believe that such studies are unlikely to be published. This can lead to publication bias.

8. In response to the incentive structure, researchers can engage in gaming the system by manipulating citation metrics.

9. The fraud triangle identifies three factors that together lead to research misconduct: incentives, opportunity and rationalisation.

    (a) the personal and professional rewards from novel and exciting findings provide the motivation for misconduct.

    (b) opportunity is provided by the options for flexibility (cheating) during the conduct of research, and the low likelihood of being caught.

    (c) behavioural biases provide mechanisms through which well-motivated individuals can rationalise their engagement in data falsification and questionable research practices.

10. Humans have a capacity for self-deception that enables them to be dishonest, while believing that they are not doing harm. Many unconscious biases assist this process.

11. A belief that they are being treated unfairly by the research system can also help researchers justify misbehaviours.

12. Some researchers feel that, because others cheat without being caught, they need to do likewise to avoid being left behind.

13. Conflict of interest can bias judgement during the conduct of research. Little account is taken of the impact that declared conflict of interest may have on study findings.

THE FINDINGS IN PERSPECTIVE

This negative assessment of research needs to be put into perspective. Many clinical trials and systematic reviews are of high quality, and they have identified effective treatments for a host of diseases including cancer, heart disease, stroke and diabetes [1–3]. These advances should be celebrated as examples of what high quality research can achieve; they set the standard that all researchers should strive to emulate.

In the main, researchers do not set out to conduct biased or poor quality studies. Most scientists consider themselves honest, and follow a research career with the aim of 'doing good work. . . and making a genuine and lasting contribution' [4]. They are motivated partly by curiosity and a desire to find out how things work, and also by the esteem of their peers [5]. Belief in the value of the work they do and maintaining 'the standards of the scientific process' are central to their professional behaviour [6]. However, the way the research environment is organised, its structures and pressures lead some individuals to engage in misconduct. The prevention of poor quality and wasted research will require major changes in the behaviour of the individuals and institutions that sponsor, conduct and publish medical research.

REFERENCES

1. Siegel, R.L., Miller, K.D., and Jemal, A. (2016). Cancer statistics, 2016. *CA Cancer J. Clin.* 66: 7–30.

2. Nathan, D.M. (2015). Diabetes: advances in diagnosis and treatment. *JAMA* 314: 1052–1062.

3. Collins, R., Reith, C., Emberson, J. et al. (2016). Interpretation of the evidence for the efficacy and safety of statin therapy. *Lancet* 388: 2532–2561.

4. Munafo, M.R. (2019). Commentary on Gorman (2019): publication procedures are only part of the solution. *Addiction* 114: 1487–1488.

5. Franck, G. (2015). The wage of fame: how non-epistemic motives have enabled the phenomenal success of modern science. *Gerontology* 61: 89–94.

6. Ryan, J. (2014). The work motivation of research scientists and its effect on research performance. *R&D Manag.* 44: 355–369.

Appendix 2: Initiatives to Improve the Quality of Research

This appendix reviews initiatives that have been proposed to redress poorly reported, misleading and wasted research. They are organised in four categories: the research environment; research transparency; research oversight and research integrity. The list is long and its constituents are diverse, indicating a widespread recognition of the need for change and the large number of issues to be addressed. Most of these initiatives could be helpful, although some will be challenging to implement. A few are included for completeness even though they are unlikely to be helpful.

CHANGE THE RESEARCH ENVIRONMENT

The malign effects of hypercompetition, pressure to publish, perverse incentives and the rhetoric of excellence are widely recognised. The scientific community has responded with several important initiatives to address them [1–5].

Value Negative Findings

Trials with negative findings are at an increased risk of not being published. This may be one explanation for the gradual disappearance

Evidence in Medicine: The Common Flaws, Why They Occur and How to Prevent Them, First Edition. Iain K Crombie.
© 2021 John Wiley & Sons Ltd. Published 2021 by John Wiley & Sons Ltd.

of negative findings from the scientific literature [6]. Concern about this led publishers to establish several journals dedicated to negative findings [7, 8]. In addition open access journals, such as Plos One and F1000 Research, welcome negative findings.

The World Medical Association, the International Committee of Medical Journal Editors and the Committee on Publication Ethics place responsibility for the publication of negative findings on journal editors [9]. Some journals have published editorials stating a willingness to publish negative findings [10], although the issue is still being discussed [9]. To facilitate the publication of negative findings, Earp and Wilkinson have suggested that journal editors could use a simple symmetry test [11]. If a paper has positive findings, they should ask whether they would accept an identical paper with negative findings. Similarly, for a paper with negative findings, would they have published it if the findings were positive? At the heart of this test lie two questions: does the study address an important issue, and is the methodology adequate to provide a meaningful answer. Earp and Wilkinson recommend that this test be added as a compulsory item in the editorial review process [11].

Solutions to the problem of unpublished studies with negative findings do not only lie with medical journals; the researchers, funding agencies, research institutions, regulatory agencies and legislators all have a role [12]. To assist their endeavours, Meerpohl and colleagues have produced detailed recommendations for each of these stakeholders [12]. They are intended to promote the dissemination of all findings and to ensure that study data are made available to other researchers.

Change Research Assessment

A very high value is placed on exciting new results [3, 5], providing the incentive to engineer such findings [13–16]. Shifting the emphasis from sensational findings to the importance of the research question, and to the rigour of the methodology, would promote rigorous research [17]. One way to achieve this would be to change research assessment, the system for assessing an individual's research standing, as this 'powerfully influences scientists' behaviour' [18].

Research assessment predominantly uses publication metrics, such as the publication in a high quality journal and the frequency with which papers are cited by other articles. The hiring, promotion and tenure of researchers are determined by these criteria [18]. This process is thought to be 'jeopardizing the integrity of the scientific literature' [19]. The assessment system may have the unintended consequence of encouraging underpowered studies with spuriously significant findings [3]. It may also lead to a data fabrication, and to a variety of questionable research practices.

The San Francisco Declaration On Research Assessment (DORA) was an important step towards changing the present methods of research evaluation [20]. It states that journal impact factors should not be used to assess the quality of a research article, for the hiring or promotion of individuals, or the awarding of research grants. Instead the research should be assessed on its own merits. Since its launch in 2012, many journals, funding bodies and professional societies have implemented proposals to reduce the use or prominence of impact factors [21]. Despite the DORA initiative, journal impact factors are still widely used [22–24].

As the present metrics are counterproductive, finding alternative measures would seem a high priority: 'If rigorous, innovative studies of significant issues and publication of valid, reproducible results are desired, the best way to achieve those objectives is to explicitly evaluate and reward scientists based on those criteria' [19]. The Open Science movement strongly supports rewarding scientists for the quality of their research [25] and participating in data sharing [26]. A formal statement on valuing science, the Hong Kong Principles for assessing researchers, was developed following The 2019 World Conferences on Research Integrity [27]. Its five principles widen the scope of assessment from the use of publication metrics, to include the importance of the research question, the rigour of the methods and the publishing of negative findings, as well as the practices of open science, such as data sharing [27]. A novel idea is to measure the impact of a research study by its uptake on social media, as well as by traditional citation measures. Finally they suggest that activities other than publications, such as peer review, mentoring and social outreach, should be included in the assessment process.

Worldwide implementation of these proposals would transform research assessment and, in doing so, the quality of research.

Some care may be needed to ensure researchers do not devise strategies to manipulate any new criteria. Many techniques have been used to artificially inflate citation metrics [28], and researchers are likely to be equally inventive with any new criteria. Uptake by social media and social outreach activities might be particularly susceptible to such gaming.

Improve Training

Although there is a wealth of easily accessible guidance on the conduct of trials, systematic reviews and data analysis, the use of poorly described or inadequate methods is common [29]. Given the extent of poor quality research, it is hard to avoid the conclusion that many researchers do not know how to design and conduct high quality studies. An editorial in 1994 by Doug Altman [30] described the problem: 'researchers feel compelled for career reasons to carry out research that they are ill equipped to perform, and nobody stops them'. The point was recently restated: 'young clinicians are encouraged to carry out and publish research, often without adequate research training or supervision' [31].

Recognition that the methodological expertise of some researchers is weak has led several authors to recommend that further training should be given [32–37]. The World Medical Association Declaration of Helsinki states that 'Medical research involving human subjects must be conducted only by individuals with the appropriate ethics and scientific education, training and qualifications' [38]. At present there is no 'required educational background or defined set of competencies' for those conducting clinical research [39]. Several groups have developed core competencies for clinical research to help define the types of training needed [40–42]. One good example of training is that provided by the Cochrane Collaboration for the conduct of systematic reviews. Its educational activities include online courses, videos, webinars, learning events, and guides and handbooks [43]. Although formal training is essential, it may be insufficient on its own: trainees also require effective mentorship [44] within a productive research environment [45].

Initiatives to improve the expertise of researchers face several challenges. The individuals who need training will have to be identified and motivated to engage in educational activities. There may be some reluctance among established researchers to accept that they need to participate. The training is likely to involve didactic and experiential learning, and will need the support of supervisors or mentors. Training will need to be recognised as a legitimate activity, with appropriate time set aside for both trainee and trainer. Developing suitable and effective teaching materials is possibly the most difficult task. The combination of high quality training, mentorship, a supportive research environment and protected time may be difficult to achieve.

Certificates of Research Competence

To ensure that the training is adequate and effective, a system of certification of clinical researchers has been proposed [46]. Similarly it has been suggested that academics supervising research should hold a licence to supervise [47]. A certificate of competence, possibly based on the publication of previous relevant high quality studies, would enable skilled researchers to continue working. Junior researchers would work towards accreditation by compiling evidence of competence in aspects of the study design and conduct during involvement in a study. With sufficient experience these researchers could progress to receive the certificate of competence. Attainment of core competencies is a prerequisite for the practice of medicine. Give the current deplorable state of evidence, it might seem sensible to have a similar system for medical research.

Trial Forge

Trial Forge is an international collaboration that compiles and disseminates guidance on trial conduct to improve quality and make the process more efficient [48]. It aims to be the go-to site for trial methodology. Evidence packs and videos on techniques for recruitment and retention can be accessed from its website (https://www. trialforge.org/trial-forge-resources). It also promotes research on effective ways to design, run, analyse and report trials.

PRECIS-2

PRECIS-2 is a validated tool to help researchers design 'trials that are fit for purpose' [49]. Developed by an international team of over 80 experts, it guides researchers through the main stages of trials, such as setting the eligibility criteria, methods for participant recruitment, the expertise and resources needed, the choice of outcome measures and the methods of follow-up [49]. The tool will also help ensure that trials are designed and conducted to provide results that are relevant to both clinicians and patients.

INCREASE RESEARCH TRANSPARENCY

Many initiatives, dating over several decades, have been proposed to make the conduct of research more visible, and thus more open to scrutiny. This section briefly describes three overlapping initiatives: data sharing, Open Science and the RIAT initiative.

Data Sharing

The suggestion that the raw data from studies should be shared with other interested researchers was made over 40 years ago [50]. Recent initiatives from the US Institute of Medicine, the European Medicines Agency, pharmaceutical companies and the International Committee of Medical Journal Editors have supported the sharing of data from clinical trials [51–53]. Providing other research groups with trials data could have two important benefits. A reanalysis would confirm, or refute, the published findings, providing an assurance of research quality [54]. Further analyses might also reveal 'that new nuggets of useful data are lying there, previously unseen' [55].

Data sharing is seen as an ethical and scientific imperative [56]. Its value was clearly seen during the Covid 19 pandemic, with researchers using infrastructure platforms to share their data prior to formal publication [57]. Although there are technical and financial issues to resolve, most researchers and research institutions are strongly supportive of this initiative [58]. But some concerns have been expressed about data sharing. A research group who were not involved in the study might not fully understand the decisions taken during data collection and processing [55]. Other issues include patient data privacy, insufficient recognition of the data originators' contribution [59], and multiple testing that results in spuriously positive findings [60].

The FAIR principles for data stewardship have been developed to facilitate data sharing, stressing data sets should be Findable, Accessible, Interoperable and Reusable [61]. In a separate initiative a taskforce outlined 10 principles and 50 recommendations to cover the fundamental requirements of data sharing for clinical trials [62]. The experience of the YODA project in sharing data illustrates the many challenges for this activity [63].

At present the rates of data sharing are low, which is unsurprising given the many hurdles to overcome and the paucity of evidence-based incentives with which to promote its uptake [64]. As Rockhold and colleagues commented, the question is not 'whether data should be shared, but rather how and when responsible methods for doing so can be ushered in' [59]. Data sharing is an important initiative, but its full value will only be realised if it is adequately resourced. The creation of a new funding stream, which incorporated appropriate principles and safeguards, would prove a worthwhile investment.

Open Science

Open Science is a collection of initiatives that 'promote openness, integrity, and reproducibility in research' [26]. To support this movement a set of Transparency and Openness Promotion (TOP) Guidelines were produced, which journals could include in their instructions to authors [65]. The International Committee of Medical Journal Editors has issued its own data sharing statement [52].

Open Science encourages sharing of data and research materials, pre-registration of study methods, the conduct of replication studies, open access publishing and improved methods of peer review [26]. One aim is to reduce questionable practices, such as manipulated statistical analysis and selective outcome reporting, by increasing transparency about the hypotheses being tested, the methods being used and the statistical analyses [25, 26]. If widely implemented, Open Science will enable reanalysis and replication of selected studies [26, 66]. At present, Open Science relies on altruistic behaviour by researchers willing to take on the tasks of documenting and archiving all study materials for others to use [66]. To support them in this endeavour Barend Mons has suggested that 5% of the money allocated to research should be used to ensure that data are reusable [67]. Ensuring that researchers receive an appropriate form of academic credit might also increase the compliance with this important movement.

The RIAT Initiative

Concerns about the potential impact of unpublished and misreported studies led to the RIAT initiative (Restoring Invisible and Abandoned Trials) [68]. Funding enabled the establishment of a RIAT Support Centre to assist researchers in accessing and reanalysing unpublished data [69]. Trials of two treatments widely used for vomiting in pregnancy [70, 71], and one for major depression in adolescence [72], have been successfully evaluated. Careful reanalysis of the full data shows the original claims for effectiveness to be incorrect, or unwarranted because of high risk of bias [70–72]. Further assessments of published trials are underway. This initiative clearly demonstrates the value of data sharing, and the need for a funding stream to support the reanalysis of other trials.

QUALITY OF TRIAL METHODOLOGY

The CONSORT Statement for Trials

Concerns about the poor reporting of clinical trial methods and results led to the creation of the CONSORT statement in 1996 (Consolidated Standards of Reporting Trials) [73]. This identifies the items that should be addressed in trial reports. The statement was revised and expanded in 2001 and 2010, and currently lists 25 items. It is accompanied by helpful explanations of exactly what is required and why it is important [74]. In addition, several extensions have been made to the statement to deal with specific issues such as the reporting of harms, the writing of abstracts and the description of non-pharmacological interventions [75].

Adherence to the CONSORT statement is often poor, with many items not being reported [76, 77]. Even the items most important for assessing risk of bias are often inadequately described: an overview of over 20,000 trials found that in 49% of trials, the risk of bias for the generation of the randomisation could not be assessed [78]. Similarly, allocation concealment was unclear in 58% of trials, blinding of outcome assessment in 31% and incomplete outcome data in 25%. Over time, 1986 to 2014, the proportion of trials with unclear sequence generation and allocation concealment greatly reduced, but the falls for blinding and incomplete assessment were much smaller [78]. The problem has been ameliorated but not solved.

The CONSORT statement has been endorsed by the World Association of Medical Editors, the International Committee of Medical Journal Editors (ICMJE), and the Council of Science Editors [79]. However many journals may not follow this recommendation. Surveys of high impact journals found that in 2003 only 22% mentioned the statement in their instructions to authors, but that this had increased to 63% by 2014 [80]. Journals with lower impact factors may be less likely to endorse CONSORT [81]. In addition some journals may endorse CONSORT but not enforce it: a survey of surgical journals revealed that while 42% mentioned it, only 33% required it [81]

The SPIRIT 2013 Statement for Study Protocols

Protocols for clinical trials often omit important details such as the primary outcome and the sample size calculation [82]. The SPIRIT initiative (Standard Protocol Items: Recommendations for Interventional Trials) was launched in 2007 to improve the quality of protocols. Researchers were encouraged to provide a detailed description of the study methods and the planned statistical analysis. The statement was updated in 2013 to provide a checklist of 33 essential items to be presented in protocols [83]. A companion paper gives helpful guidance on what should be included under each heading [84].

The protocol can serve an important role in research transparency, by providing fuller details of the rationale for the trial and of the methods to be used. Comparison of the protocol with the final published paper can reveal changes to the study design, such as switching outcome measures, or modifications to the planned analysis [85]. Although making protocols publicly available is strongly encouraged, most trials protocols are not easily accessible [86]. This is an important challenge to Open Science.

Reporting the Statistical Analysis: The SAMPL Guidelines

Errors are common 'in the application, analysis, interpretation, or reporting of statistics' [87]. Despite the availability of a host of textbooks on medical statistics, these problems persist. Over 40 years ago, O'Fallen and colleagues suggested that reporting standards should be developed for authors and be enforced by reviewers and editorial boards [50]. Many medical journals provide statistical guidelines for authors and, partly based on these, the SAMPL Guidelines (Statistical Analyses and Methods in the Published Literature) were prepared. These provide clear advice for the reporting of statistical analyses for authors, journal editors and reviewers [87].

Reporting Harms

Recognition that adverse events are frequently under-reported in published clinical trials led a multidisciplinary group to meet in May 2003. They subsequently produced an Extension to the CONSORT statement to improve the reporting of harms [88]. Despite this, harms continue to be poorly reported in published papers [89–92]. One suggestion is that medical journals could require that published reports explicitly follow the CONSORT recommendations on harms [90, 93]. In addition some authors recommend that unpublished data from clinical trial registries and regulatory bodies should be searched to ensure that reporting is complete [89, 92]. Poor reporting of harms is a continuing problem, which could lead to bias in the assessment of the benefit to harm ratio of treatments.

Reporting Trial Findings

Concerns about the number of unpublished trials led the European Union, in 2004, to require that all trials of medicinal products conducted in an EU country must post their results on the European Union Clinical Trials Register within one year of study completion [94]. In 2015, the World Health Organisation updated its 2005 statement on trial reporting, reaffirming the ethical imperative of the timely reporting of clinical trials [95]. In the US, the Food and Drugs Administration passed a law in 2007 that certain categories of clinical trials had to publish their findings on the website http://ClinicalTrials.gov within 12 months of completion of the study [96]. The penalty for failure to do so was a fine of up to $10,000 for each day of delay [97]. All the necessary supporting procedure for registration were not in place until 2017, at which point a Final Rule came into effect, mandating the prompt reporting of trials [96].

Despite these statements the reporting of trials remains unsatisfactory. A recent analysis of studies in the EU Clinical trials Register found that only one half of the trials had reported within 12 months of their scheduled completion [94]. An analysis of compliance with the US Food and Drugs Administration's 2007 Act found that only 13% of trials had reported within 12 months [97]. A more recent analysis of the impact of the 2017 New Rule found that only 41% reported their results within one year [96]. The conclusion drawn from the US and the EU experiences is that 'trial reporting will only improve when regulators routinely impose fines and other sanctions' on those who do not comply [96].

TRIAL REGISTRATION

The establishment of mechanisms for prospective trial registration has been described as 'the single most valuable tool we have to ensure unbiased reporting' [98]. The need for a register of all clinical trials was recognised in the 1970s, and became an ethical imperative in the early years of the twenty-first century [99]. The triggering event was the launch of the trial registration policy by the International Committee of Medical Journal Editors in September 2004 [100]. This proposed that all trials should be registered, so that key features of the study design would be described before the trial began. Any subsequent modifications to the study design would also be recorded. A searchable database of all ongoing and completed trials [100] would enable the detection of scientific misconduct, such as non-publication of findings, changing the primary outcome or reporting outcomes that had not been pre-specified [99].

Trial registration is emphasised in the CONSORT and SPIRIT statements and is required by many funding bodies, research ethics committees and the International Committee of Medical Journal Editors [101]. Several international registers have been established (e.g. http://ClinicalTrials.gov and the ISRCTN registry) [99, 100]. Their use is recommended or mandated by governments and funding bodies around the world and is a prerequisite for publication in many leading medical journals.

Enforcement of Trial Registration

Enforcement of pre-registration of trials has been proposed because current compliance is unsatisfactory [100]. A recent study found that, although 53% had been registered, only one trial in five had been registered prospectively [102]. Even among the prestigious high impact journals only about 70% of published trials were registered prospectively [103, 104]. This is concerning because trials that have not been registered, on average, report larger effect sizes than registered ones [105, 106].

One suggestion for improving prospective registration is to make it a condition of the award of ethical approval, a method that is popular among researchers [107]. The United Kingdom has required registration as a condition of a favourable ethical opinion since 2013, but a recent study found that only 80% of clinical trials had been registered [108]. The authors of that report suggest that some method of audit of registration, combined with sanctions, might be needed to achieve 100% registration.

REPORTING OF THE METHODS
OF SYSTEMATIC REVIEWS

The PRISMA statement (Preferred Reporting Items for Systematic reviews and Meta-Analyses) was published in 2009 [109]. It specifies 27 items that should be addressed, and provides a flow diagram to describe the stages of identification and selection of trials to be included in the review. The PRISMA statement is an update of an earlier statement (QUOROM: QUality Of Reporting Of Meta-analyses) and was intended to improve the presentation of 'what was planned, done, and found in a systematic review' [109]. An extension to the original statement focused on the structure of the abstract and the items to be included in it [110]. This was needed because many abstracts were inadequate: for example, the direction of effect (whether the treatment was beneficial or harmful) was often unclear. More recently a further extension, dealing with the reporting of harms, was published [111].

Providing guidance is an important step forward, but this does not mean that researchers always follow it. One recent assessment found that only one third of systematic reviews adhered to at least 10 of the 27 items on the PRISMA statement [112]. Another showed that the rationale for the study and the sources searched were well described in 85% of reviews, the eligibility criteria in 77%, a detailed search strategy in 50% and only 6% mentioned a registered or published protocol [113]. Possibly the methods to ensure the registration and full reporting of clinical trials could be adapted to cover systematic reviews.

Registration of Protocols of Systematic Reviews

Pre-registration of protocols of systematic reviews was a key recommendation of the PRISMA statement [114]. The aims were 'to reduce unplanned duplication of systematic reviews and to provide transparency of the review process' [114]. The drive to registration was aided by the launch, in February 2011, of PROSPERO, an international register of the protocols of systematic reviews [115]. Leading organisations, such as the Cochrane Collaboration and the US Agency for Heathcare Research and Quality, require that the protocol should be registered or published before a systematic review is conducted. To ensure the protocols are of high quality, guidance on their contents was provided in the PRISMA-P statement in 2015 [116]. A helpful companion paper to PRISMA-P gives a full description of the main items to be addressed in a protocol and explains why these are important [117].

From a slow start, the rate of registration quickly increased, so that by the beginning of 2018 an estimated 30,000 reviews had been registered [115]. Compared to the 20,000 reviews that are published each year [118], the cumulative total of 30,000 appears modest. However, if the rate of registration continues to accelerate, a large proportion of reviews could be registered. This would be aided if funding bodies and medical journals made pre-registration mandatory. Research using the PROSPERO register showed that reviews that are prospectively registered were of higher quality than unregistered ones [119, 120], and reported their methods in more detail [121].

The registration scheme facilitates the investigation of questionable practices. One study found that for 32% of registered reviews, the primary outcome was changed or omitted from protocol to publication [122]. Another study confirmed frequent inconsistencies in the primary outcome, but also found changes in the statistical analysis in 52% of reviews [123]. The position is even worse for reviews that are not conducted through the Cochrane Collaboration: in almost all (92%) the protocol and final publication have differences in methods, and 49% of these inconsistencies were considered major. Only 7% of studies gave an explanation for the differences [124]. There is a need for some system of checking that the registered methods of systematic reviews are consistent with those reported in the published papers.

INCREASING ACCESS TO AND USE OF REPORTING GUIDELINES

EQUATOR and Reporting Guidelines

The EQUATOR Network (Enhancing the QUAlity and Transparency Of health Research) has collated the CONSORT, SPIRIT and PRISMA statements, together with similar guidelines for other study designs, to improve the reporting of health research [125]. Officially launched in 2008, it provides a free online resource of reporting guidelines. As of May 2020 it contained 428 reporting guidelines (https://www.equator-network.org), and an international team is constantly updating the list.

Interventions to Promote Guideline Use

Despite the easy availability of reporting guidelines, evaluations of published studies show that their use is often suboptimal [126]. As a result, many interventions have been designed to improve this [127]. In total 31 initiatives have been targeted at different aspects of guideline use, such as increasing access, provision of training, monitoring with feedback, and involving experts. Only four of these interventions had been evaluated in trials, with most being assessed in observational studies. Those evaluated in trials have produced mixed results. A web-based tool developed to promote adherence to the CONSORT statement was tested and found to be ineffective [128]. However, the inclusion of a statistician with experience of CONSORT in the peer review process led to more complete reporting of the trial methods [129]. The authors of the scoping review reported that 'Additional research is needed to assess the effectiveness of many of these interventions' [127].

IMPLEMENT VIGOROUS RESEARCH OVERSIGHT

Strengthen Peer Review

Effective peer review is seen as central to tackling the poor quality of medical research [130, 131]. A system of research oversight that detected methodological flaws, and data manipulation, could deter misconduct. Concerns have been expressed about the current effectiveness of peer review [132]. A recent editorial in a leading journal commented that peer review 'is of questionable value and could offer false reassurance' [133]. Part of the problem is that reviewers focus more on whether a finding would be important if it were true, than in assessing whether the claim could be true [134].

Several suggestions have been made to improve peer review. One is to require that researchers should provide the full study protocol when submitting a trial manuscript for publication [135]. This would provide more detailed information on the study methods. Comparing the protocol and the submitted manuscript could detect discrepancies such as outcome switching, or unplanned subgroup analyses. Wicherts has expanded on this to suggest that as well as the study protocol, reviewers should be given the research materials (e.g. questionnaires) and the complete data set [136]. This would enable a fuller investigation of potential misconduct, but would place a substantial extra burden on the reviewer.

Improving the skills of editors and peer reviewers could also improve peer review. Moher and Altman [130] have suggested that training in a set of core competences should be provided for peer reviewers and journal editors. This could be funded by a small levy, the authors suggest 0.1% of the expenditure of research funders and publishers. A complementary approach would be to use a trial methodologist, who would focus exclusively on technical issues likely to introduce bias, such as allocation concealment [137]. Another suggestion is to provide reviewers with a set of objective criteria to assess the quality of the methods and statistical analysis [131]. An extension of this proposal is to require that authors explain the rationale for their statistical analyses, which the reviewers should evaluate [138]. Finally, specialist statistical reviewers have been shown to improve the quality of research papers [139, 140]. Many journals currently use statistical reviewers, but this could be extended to all journals. Large numbers of experienced statisticians would be needed to provide this service, and it is far from clear that this is feasible at present.

Alternative Forms of Peer Review

A radical alternative to conventional peer review would be to base the decision whether to publish a paper on the research question, the rationale for the study and the detailed methodology. This has been termed results-blind review [141], in which the decision on paper acceptance is based on the importance of the research question and the rigour of the study design. This approach has been formalised in the Registered Report; researchers submit details of the proposed research (study rationale, methods and analysis plan) before collecting any data. The editorial team and the reviewers are not swayed by an exciting new result, and researchers have no incentive to massage their data to produce one. Instead the emphasis is placed on important research questions and high quality, robust methods. Over 200 journals have adopted this approach [142, 143], which could improve research quality and increase the frequency with which non-significant findings are published [66].

The British Journal of Anaesthetics is currently testing another novel approach in which the journal editor invites an independent specialist to write a Discussion section based on the protocol, methods, results and the raw data [144, 145]. The original discussion is withheld. At present, the authors 'discuss their own findings, point out their own shortcomings, and selectively review the existing literature' [146]. An independent discussion could provide a more objective and balanced assessment of the findings and prevent spin, over-interpretation of results and the understatement of limitations. The drawback is the additional demand placed on expert reviewers [146], although this could be overcome by ensuring that the second discussion counts as a publication [145].

Reward Peer Reviewers

The careful appraisal of a paper is time consuming but carries little benefit to the reviewer, and indeed diverts efforts away from doing research. This may explain why, in a time of hypercompetition, journals are finding it difficult to recruit reviewers [147]. Zietman has suggested that the review should be published alongside the article, giving credit to the reviewers for their efforts [148]. It might also provide the reviewer with an incentive to produce a high quality review.

Another possible solution is the Publons initiative. This provides an online platform where those invited to carry out a review can have it posted anonymously on the Publons website [149]. Many leading publishers have endorsed Publons, and the initiative appears popular with reviewers [149, 150]. The system records the reviews that have been undertaken and publishes lists of the top reviewers. One group has suggested that points could be awarded for reviews, which could subsequently be traded for a reduction in the fees charged for publication in open access journals [151]. If high quality peer reviews were rewarded in ways that benefitted their career prospects, researchers would be more willing to devote time to it.

Audit Trial Publication

To prevent publication bias, the European Union [94], the US Food and Drugs Administration [96] and the World Health Organisation [95] propose that all trials should be reported one year after the proposed study's completion date. Goldacre suggested that this be audited, locally and centrally, and the data used to identify individuals and institutions who fail to report trial findings [152]. This information could subsequently be published to incentivise the reporting of findings in a timely manner. To facilitate this type of audit, DeVito and colleagues developed an automated trial tracker that monitored all trials registered on http://ClinicalTrials.gov [153]. The researchers overcame several administrative and technical difficulties, and successfully identified the studies that were unpublished or published late. This approach could be extended to other clinical trial registries, but will require a combination of commitment and interpersonal and technical skills.

Kolstoe and colleagues investigated a different method. They realised that 'ethical review bodies are well placed to check trial reporting', and could take the lead in auditing publication of findings [154]. Pilot testing showed the method was feasible, and that one researcher could review 116 projects in one year. This approach could be used when administrative or technical hurdles preclude the use of an automated trial tracker. Koltoe et al.'s article included a commentary from Janet Wisely, who raised concerns about the resources required for the auditing and the lack sanctions for transgression [154]. These are important issues.

Monitor for Selective Outcome Reporting

Differences are often seen in the primary and secondary outcomes described at the start of a trial and those in the final manuscript of findings. Regularly checking published studies against the details in international trial registers could deter individuals from selective outcome reporting [155]. The aim is to prevent 'differing definitions being used and only the most favourable result being reported' [156]. The COMPare Project evaluated outcome reporting for trials published in four leading journals over a four-month period; it established that many pre-specified outcomes languished unreported, and many unspecified outcomes were added [157]. If the risk of detection were greater, researchers might be less willing to make these changes. Applying sanctions, such as rejecting papers found to have unexplained changes in outcomes [158], or even blacklisting of authors [159], could increase the deterrence effect. To enable comparisons to be made, the outcomes need to be specified in detail at registration, giving the time point and the exact metric used [156, 160].

The challenge of this approach is the workload, with one group calculating that some 200 trials would need to be assessed each day [157]. These authors recognise that medical journals do not have the resources to conduct these checks in house, and suggest that expert groups could be involved. Another suggestion is that funding bodies or Research Ethics Committees could carry out this work [159]. These proposals would all require skilled individuals willing to devote time to the task. It is unclear whether Research Ethics Committees would agree to take on this additional task: they have many other important tasks to complete.

Preprints and Pre-Publication Review

Online repositories (preprint servers) have been established so that researchers can post drafts of their papers prior to publication in a peer-reviewed journal. This enables more rapid dissemination of findings [161] and provides an opportunity to detect and remedy errors before formal publication [162]. Rapid communication of findings was important during the Zika and Ebola outbreaks [163], and the 2020 Covid 19 pandemic witnessed 'the powerful role preprints can have during public health crises because of the timeliness with which they can disseminate new information' [164].

For most medical research, progress is slow and careful reflection on findings is recommended [165]. One limitation of preprints is that poor research, which has not undergone formal peer review, could harm patients [166]. Reviews of preprints could identify substandard research, but in practice this benefit may not be realised. While the number of manuscripts posted on preprint servers is increasing rapidly, the frequency of online comments, which was small to start with, is declining [167]. Preprints may facilitate rapid dissemination, but concerns about their quality remain [168].

Post-Publication Review

The letters columns of journals provide a forum for criticisms of published papers [169]. This can alert readers to deficiencies in the studies, but the approach has limitations. Journals often do not publish such letters, and when they do, the average interval between the paper and the critical comments is three months [170]. Although authors are encouraged to respond to these criticisms, they often do not [171].

As well as publishing letters, some journals accept or invite commentaries on selected papers. An evaluation 130,000 clinical research studies revealed that only 5% had some form of published discussion (letter or commentary) [172]. Most of the commentaries had a supportive tone, rather than serving 'as a prominent mechanism for critical appraisal'.

Online platforms, such as ScienceOpen or PubPeer, allow any reader to post a comment on a paper [151]. Many corrections to articles, and some retractions, have resulted from criticisms reported in online platforms in the public domain [173]. Some authors have raised concerns about the competence of the reviewers, who may or may not have expertise in the relevant field [174]. Despite the ease of access, and the enthusiasm of some commentators [151, 175], the uptake of the opportunity to review is not great: one platform that had hosted such commentaries was discontinued due to insufficient interest [176]. Two factors, the absence of academic rewards for posting comments, and fear of possible retribution, may discourage researchers from commenting [175]. Recognition of post-publication review in research assessment exercises might be one way to increase its uptake.

PROMOTE RESEARCH INTEGRITY

National Level Initiatives

Concerns in the US about high-profile cases of research misconduct in the 1970s and 1980s led to the creation of the Office of Scientific Integrity, and subsequently to the Office of Research Integrity in 1993 [177]. It promotes good practice, provides guidance on research misconduct, and investigates thoroughly cases of suspected fraud. The World Conferences on Research Integrity, which began in 2007, have supported efforts in many countries to develop their own strategies [178]. The 2nd World Congress in 2010 resulted in the promulgation of the Singapore statement on research integrity [179], which forms the basis of many national and international codes of conduct [180]. Most universities in the United States [181], Canada [182] and many European countries, particularly in Western Europe, have policies on research integrity [183–187].

Despite many years of efforts to promote the responsible conduct of research, serious misconduct remains a problem [188]. Although policies on research integrity exist in many countries, they differ in the way they define terms and proposed actions to prevent misconduct [189]. The Bonn PRINTEGER Statement (Promoting Integrity as an Integral Dimension of Excellence in Research) identifies 12 key actions that research institutions could take to improve integrity [190]. These cover establishing an integrity committee, implementing quality assurance procedures and providing safe and effective channels for whistleblowing. But they also include appointing an ombudsperson, having transparency about all procedures, implementing wise incentive management and having an improved work environment. Rather than just focusing on surveillance, detection and punishment, integrity programmes should also promote 'care and concern for the research environment' [191].

Two other proposals could increase the attention institutions give to research integrity. One way to encourage this would be to include the quality of a university's research integrity programme in the evaluation of its research performance [192]. (Many countries have a formal assessment of the research outputs of their universities.) The other approach would make high quality training in research integrity in universities a condition of obtaining research funding [193]. Attendance at courses on the responsible conduct of research would be mandatory and frequent, and could cover training of trainers and as well as research integrity. The aim should be to ensure that integrity policies were highly visible and that all researchers were aware of the procedures for raising concerns [194]. Institutions would also have to take appropriate steps to create a culture of honesty and responsible behaviour. University prestige and research funding could be powerful levers for behaviour change.

Training in Research Integrity

Training programmes to promote integrity are widespread, but vary substantially in content, teaching methods and quality [188, 195]. Courses are often outsourced or run online, 'which underscores the low priority of this instruction' [196]. The effectiveness of online courses is in doubt and a key element of training, discussions between supervisor and trainee, may seldom take place [197]. Another matter of concern, is whether the funding for these initiatives is adequate [195]. Finally many courses do not provide information on key topics, such as how to deal with a senior colleague when raising misconduct issues [196].

A major challenge for integrity training is the paucity of evidence for effective approaches to preventing misconduct: a recent Cochrane review concluded that 'the effects of training in responsible conduct of research on reducing research misconduct are uncertain' [198]. A previous study drew a similar conclusion that, despite its long history, there was 'minimal evidence for effectiveness' [199]. Further, researchers themselves have 'little confidence in the ability of ethics training to improve research integrity' [200]. This problem was highlighted by a recent trial that found that the training was counterproductive: it served only to increase researchers' ability to rationalise their misbehaviour [201]. Clearly, there is a need for additional approaches to improving research integrity [195]. Possibly, as Satalkar and Shaw suggest, training will have little impact 'unless it is coupled with the creation of research culture where raising concerns is a standard practice of scientific and research activities' [202].

Monitor Data Quality

Guidelines on good clinical practice require that the data collected be subjected to some form of verification to ensure their integrity [203]. Source data verification is a process in which the data collected during a trial is compared with the details recorded in the original sources. Routine auditing of data to check validity is commonly used in trials sponsored by the pharmaceutical industry, but has been less used in other types of funded research [204, 205]. Conducting 100% source data verification can be expensive, and it has been suggested that the cost is not justified by the improvements in data quality [205]. Recently, a more selective approach, termed risk-based monitoring, has been suggested by regulatory authorities [203]. Rather than auditing all of the data for all trials, more attention could be given to those trials that might pose a high risk to participants. Additionally measurements that are critical to the findings, for example the outcome measure and the reporting of adverse effects, could be targeted.

Statistical methods provide a way to identify data fraud and fabrication. These look for strange patterns in the data that would be unlikely to occur by chance. The idea behind these tests is that it is difficult to fabricate statistically plausible data [206]. People find it hard to invent truly random data; for example they show a marked preference for round numbers (such as those ending in a zero or a five) [206]. They also find it hard to falsify dates without inadvertently having clinic dates on a Sunday [207]. A variety of statistical approaches are often used [207, 208]. Even if data have been fabricated to pass some statistical tests, they are likely to fail on others (e.g. the careful cheater could ensure that the means and the variances are realistic, but they may be found out by implausible correlations between variables) [206]. These statistical techniques can be used to complement other approaches, such as risk-based monitoring: all they require is computing resource and experienced statisticians.

Promote Reporting of Fraud and Misconduct

Researchers are often reluctant to report instances of scientific misconduct [209, 210]. Recognising this, Moher and colleagues have suggested implementing a reward system for scientists who detect errors in published studies [18]. Another approach is to provide protection for those reporting researcher misconduct. Whistleblowing can result in considerable cost, so individuals might be more inclined to come forward if there were guarantees against retaliation or other harms [211, 212]. Many countries have whistleblower protection laws covering government and business [213], but these appear not to have been applied to research.

Reduce the Use of Spin

Spin is widely used and is intended to 'glamorise, promote and/or exaggerate' the rigour of research methods and the value of study findings [214]. The causes of spin lie in the incentive structure within science [215]. It has been suggested that the guidelines of the International Committee of Medical Journal Editors, which advise authors to 'emphasize the new and important aspects of your study', could encourage this practice [214].

The need for action is recognised, but strategies to reduce spin are not well developed. Researchers, research institutions, research funders, journal editors and peer reviewers are recognised to have an important role [215–218]. Some authors identify the importance of changing the perception of spin from 'commonly accepted practice to seriously detrimental practice' [215, 216]. Changing the reward system in science to one focused on high quality research that has value for patients and clinicians could also help [216]. There is a need for specific, and preferably funded, actions to address the problem. But, as Hopf and colleagues have pointed out, there is a danger that 'piecemeal solution will simply create new perverse incentives' [218].

Promote Honesty about Conflict of Interest

Most medical journals have conflict of interest policies [219], but few describe how they verify the accuracy and completeness of authors' statements, or explain the effect any conflicts may have on editorial decisions [220]. This is a problem because financial conflicts of interest are often not fully disclosed [221, 222]. Disclosure should include not just the source and amount of money received, but also the reason for the award. Currently there is a fashion for using the ambiguous phrase unpaid consultancy to describe the nature of the conflict of interest [223]. This implies that money was not received, but fails to clarify whether other gifts, such as research funding, conference fees or travel, were received. More action is needed to address conflict of interest.

One proposal to transform reporting of conflict of interest emerged from an initiative led by the US Institute of Medicine [224]. This was to create a single register in which data on conflicts of interest could be stored (in the US such information is spread across several databases). Dunn and colleagues [225] have developed this idea by suggesting an international register that is linked to all existing repositories of conflict of interest, such as universities, funding bodies and other research-related organisations. Finding the resources to support this suggestion could be difficult.

Another possibility is to make high quality conflict of interest policies a requirement for universities seeking government research funding [226]. If successful, other research funders also could adopt this approach. Failure to disclose conflict of interest could be used as a measure of professional integrity. Individuals guilty of failing to do so could be reported to their professional body.

Research Institutions and Research Integrity

One suggestion to improve research integrity is for research institutions to employ systems analogous to those which financial institutions use to prevent fraud [227]. Research institutions could put in place appropriate internal procedures, such as auditing of research protocols, the study methods and the quality of the data. A senior researcher would be tasked with reviewing and certifying the integrity of research studies. Finally, external audit would assess the standards of the research review process. This would require a major change to the conduct and culture of universities and similar institutions.

Another suggestion is that universities should invest in publication officers who could provide training on preparing manuscripts and following reporting guidelines [130]. They could also organise internal review of manuscripts before they are submitted for publication. A variation on this, which some research institutes have already adopted, is to pay for independent screening of manuscripts for problems such as errors in statistical procedures, plagiarism and the manipulation of images [228].

Criminalise Research Fraud

Although it happens rarely, researchers have been fined, given suspended sentences or sent to jail for falsifying data [229–231]. The United States has a long history of criminal prosecution for research fraud [232]. Part of the rationale for criminalisation is 'to motivate whistleblowers and deter wrongdoers' [232].

Concern has been expressed about the cost of such actions, and the difficulty of achieving the high burden of proof required in a criminal case [233]. Experience from criminology suggests that tackling 'situational factors that enhance or restrict the opportunity for illegal or imprudent behaviour' may have more practical benefit [234]. Addressing the underlying causes of research misconduct may be more rewarding than going to court.

EXAMPLES OF COORDINATED INITIATIVES

The AllTrials Campaign

The AllTrials campaign was launched in January 2013 with the title All Trials Registered/All Trials Reported [235]. It specifies what should be achieved for each of three main aims. The first aim is that the all trials are properly registered before the first patient is recruited. The other two aims are that a summary of the findings should be posted on a trials register, and that a full report of the methods and findings are made public. Fulfilling the last aim can be onerous for researchers who often only publish summaries of methods and results. Some funding bodies request comprehensive final reports, but others only require brief outlines. Provision might have to be made for additional funding to achieve this aim.

The AllTrials campaign also promotes the sharing of the data from the trial with researchers and other stakeholders. It has explored ways of enforcing and monitoring these aims, with actions identified for regulatory authorities, research funders and medical journals.

The QUEST Initiative

The QUEST initiative (Quality Ethics Open Science Translation) provides an example of a coordinated approach taken by one research institution [236]. Launched by the Berlin Institute of Health, QUEST aims to improve the quality and value of research through training and teaching. By conducting research on research, they establish the nature and scale of problems, and use this evidence to motivate engagement in educational activities. They also provide incentives to encourage responsible research practices. For example, €1,000 is given for pre-registering a study, engaging patients in research, publishing a null result, reusing data previously published by others or making study data publically available. The money can only be used to support research or for conference attendance. The aim is to improve research practices and change the scientific culture of the institution. The impacts of these initiatives are being evaluated.

The Lancet REWARD Campaign

The Lancet, a leading medical journal, launched a REWARD Campaign (REduce research Waste And Reward Diligence) [237]. Many universities, medical journals and professional bodies have signed up to this campaign. The Campaign aims to maximise research value through high quality research that focuses on the priorities of patients and clinicians, and that is fully reported. Several working groups are being convened, including those for research funders, editors and publishers and research institutions. Among seven key recommendations are that reproducible practices and studies should be rewarded; that full protocols and analysis plans should be make publicly available and that all stakeholders should ensure that research studies are registered, published and their data shared.

The UK Reproducibility Network

The UK Reproducibility Network is a good example of an initiative that aims to promote robust research by understanding the causes of poor research, then promoting training activities and disseminating best practice (www.bristol.ac.uk/psychology/research/ukrn). It works with stakeholders across science to ensure that efforts are coordinated. Examples of its areas of action include:

- the adoption of registered reports to ensure that peer review focuses on important research questions and high quality methods
- establishing a network of groups who support Open Science
- having Open Science procedures used as a criterion when recruiting staff
- encouraging editors to publish papers based on the rigour of the methods rather than to novelty of the findings, especially those which replicate previous research

REFERENCES

1. Edwards, M.A. and Roy, S. (2017). Academic research in the 21st century: maintaining scientific integrity in a climate of perverse incentives and Hypercompetition. *Environ. Eng. Sci.* 34: 51–61.
2. Alberts, B., Kirschner, M.W., Tilghman, S. et al. (2014). Rescuing US biomedical research from its systemic flaws. *Proc. Natl. Acad. Sci. U. S. A.* 111: 5773–5777.
3. Higginson, A.D. and Munafo, M.R. (2016). Current incentives for scientists lead to underpowered studies with erroneous conclusions. *PLoS Biol.* https://doi.org/10.1371/journal.pbio.1002106.

4. Joynson, C. and Leyser, O. (2015). The culture of scientific research. *F1000Res.* https://doi.org/10.12688/f1000research.6163.1.

5. Moore, S., Neylon, C., Eve, M.P. et al. (2017). "Excellence R Us": university research and the fetishisation of excellence. *Palgrave Commun.* https://doi.org/10.1057/palcomms.2016.105.

6. Fanelli, D. (2012). Negative results are disappearing from most disciplines and countries. *Scientometrics* 90: 891–904.

7. Kannan, S. and Gowri, S. (2014). Contradicting/negative results in clinical research: why (do we get these)? Why not (get these published)? Where (to publish)? *Perspect. Clin. Res.* 5: 151–153.

8. Boorman, G.A., Foster, J.R., Laast, V.A. et al. (2015). Regulatory forum opinion piece*: the value of publishing negative scientific study data. *Toxicol. Pathol.* 43: 901–906.

9. Ekmekci, P.E. (2017). An increasing problem in publication ethics: publication bias and editors' role in avoiding it. *Med. Health Care Philos.* 20: 171–178.

10. Albrecht, J., Kirtschig, G., Matin, R.N. et al. (2017). Positive about negative: no need for a pink cloud of fluff and justifications. *Br. J. Dermatol.* 177: 1–3.

11. Earp, B.D. and Wilkinson, D. (2018). The publication symmetry test: a simple editorial heuristic to combat publication bias. *J. Clin. Transl. Res.* 3: 348–350.

12. Meerpohl, J.J., Schell, L.K., Bassler, D. et al. (2015). Evidence-informed recommendations to reduce dissemination bias in clinical research: conclusions from the OPEN (overcome failure to publish nEgative fiNdings) project based on an international consensus meeting. *BMJ Open* https://doi.org/10.1136/bmjopen-2014-006666.

13. Nosek, B.A., Spies, J.R., and Motyl, M. (2012). Scientific Utopia: II. Restructuring incentives and practices to promote truth over Publishability. *Perspect. Psychol. Sci.* 7: 615–631.

14. Ware, J.J. and Munafo, M.R. (2015). Significance chasing in research practice: causes, consequences and possible solutions. *Addiction* 110: 4–8.

15. Smaldino, P.E. and McElreath, R. (2016). The natural selection of bad science. *R. Soc. Open Sci.* https://doi.org/10.1098/rsos.160384.

16. Siegel, M.G., Brand, J.C., Rossi, M.J. et al. (2018). "Publish or perish" promotes medical literature quantity over quality. *Arthroscopy* 34: 2941–2942.

17. Grimes, D.R., Bauch, C.T., and Ioannidis, J.P.A. (2018). Modelling science trustworthiness under publish or perish pressure. *R. Soc. Open Sci.* https://doi.org/10.1098/rsos.171511.

18. Moher, D., Naudet, F., Cristea, I.A. et al. (2018). Assessing scientists for hiring, promotion, and tenure. *PLoS Biol.* https://doi.org/10.1371/journal.pbio.2004089.

19. Lindner, M.D., Torralba, K.D., and Khan, N.A. (2018). Scientific productivity: an exploratory study of metrics and incentives. *PLoS One* https://doi.org/10.1371/journal.pone.0195321.

20. Anonymous (2012). San Francisco Declaration on Research Assessment. https://sfdora.org. Accessed 19 December 2019.

21. Schmid, S.L. (2017). Five years post-DORA: promoting best practices for research assessment. *Mol. Biol. Cell* 28: 2941–2944.

22. Chapman, C.A., Bicca-Marques, J.C., Calvignac-Spencer, S. et al. (2019). Games academics play and their consequences: how authorship, h-index and journal impact factors are shaping the future of academia. *Proc. Biol. Sci.* https://doi.org/10.1098/rspb.2019.2047.

23. Osterloh, M. and Frey, B.S. (2020). How to avoid borrowed plumes in academia. *Res. Policy* https://doi.org/10.1016/j.respol.2019.103831.

24. McKiernan, E.C., Schimanski, L.A., Munoz Nieves, C. et al. (2019). Use of the journal impact factor in academic review, promotion, and tenure evaluations. *elife* https://doi.org/10.7554/eLife.47338.

25. Frankenhuis, W.E. and Nettle, D. (2018). Open science is liberating and can Foster creativity. *Perspect. Psychol. Sci.* 13: 439–447.

26. Banks, G.C., Field, J.G., Oswald, F.L. et al. (2019). Answers to 18 questions about open science practices. *J. Bus. Psychol.* 34: 257–270.

27. Moher, D., Bouter, L., Kleinert, S. et al. (2020). The Hong Kong principles for assessing researchers: fostering research integrity. *PLoS Biol.* https://doi.org/10.1371/journal.pbio.3000737.

28. Ebrahim, N., Salehi, H., Embi, M.A. et al. (2013). Effective strategies for increasing citation frequency. *Int. Educ. Stud.* 6: 93–99.

29. Glasziou, P. and Chalmers, I. (2018). Research waste is still a scandal-an essay by Paul Glasziou and Iain Chalmers. *BMJ* https://doi.org/10.1136/bmj.k4645.
30. Altman, D.G. (1994). The scandal of poor medical research. *BMJ* https://doi.org/10.1136/bmj.308.6924.283.
31. Bell, R.J. (2017). What is wrong with the medical literature? *Climacteric* 20: 22–24.
32. Chalmers, I. and Glasziou, P. (2009). Avoidable waste in the production and reporting of research evidence. *Lancet* 374: 86–89.
33. Casadevall, A. and Fang, F.C. (2018). Making the scientific literature fail-safe. *J. Clin. Invest.* 128: 4243–4244.
34. Ioannidis, J.P., Fanelli, D., Dunne, D.D. et al. (2015). Meta-research: evaluation and improvement of research methods and practices. *PLoS Biol.* https://doi.org/10.1371/journal.pbio.1002264.
35. Glasziou, P., Altman, D.G., Bossuyt, P. et al. (2014). Reducing waste from incomplete or unusable reports of biomedical research. *Lancet* 383: 267–276.
36. Page, M.J. and Moher, D. (2016). Mass production of systematic reviews and meta-analyses: an exercise in mega-silliness? *Milbank Q.* 94: 515–519.
37. Li, G., Bhatt, M., Wang, M. et al. (2018). Enhancing primary reports of randomized controlled trials: three most common challenges and suggested solutions. *Proc. Natl. Acad. Sci. U. S. A.* 115: 2595–2599.
38. World Medical Association (2013). World medical association declaration of Helsinki: ethical principles for medical research involving human subjects. *JAMA* 310: 2191–2194.
39. Sonstein, S.A. and Jones, C.T. (2018). Joint task force for clinical trial competency and clinical research professional workforce development. *Front. Pharmacol.* https://doi.org/10.3389/fphar.2018.01148.
40. Forrest, C.B., Martin, D.P., Holve, E. et al. (2009). Health services research doctoral core competencies. *BMC Health Serv. Res.* https://doi.org/10.1186/1472-6963-9-107.
41. Burgess, J.F., Menachemi, N., and Maciejewski, M.L. (2018). Update on the health services research doctoral core competencies. *Health Serv. Res.* 53 (Suppl 2): 3985–4003.

42. Sonstein, S.A., Namenek Brouwer, R.J., Gluck, W. et al. (2020). Leveling the joint task force core competencies for clinical research professionals. *Ther. Innov. Regul. Sci.* 54: 1–20.
43. Anonymous (2020). Cochrane Training. https://training.cochrane.org. Accessed 2 February 2020.
44. Pfund, C., Byars-Winston, A., Branchaw, J. et al. (2016). Defining attributes and metrics of effective research mentoring relationships. *AIDS Behav.* 20: 238–248.
45. Ajjawi, R., Crampton, P.E.S., and Rees, C.E. (2018). What really matters for successful research environments? A realist synthesis. *Med. Educ.* https://doi.org/10.1111/medu.13643.
46. Lightfoot, G.D., Sanford, S.M., and Shefrin, A. (1999). Can investigator certification improve the quality of clinical research? *Qual. Manage. Health Care* 7: 31–36.
47. Bouter, L.M. (2015). Commentary: perverse incentives or rotten apples? *Account Res.* 22: 148–161.
48. Treweek, S., Altman, D.G., Bower, P. et al. (2015). Making randomised trials more efficient: report of the first meeting to discuss the trial forge platform. *Trials* https://doi.org/10.1186/s13063-015-0776-0.
49. Loudon, K., Treweek, S., Sullivan, F. et al. (2015). The PRECIS-2 tool: designing trials that are fit for purpose. *BMJ* https://doi.org/10.1136/bmj.h2147.
50. O'Fallon, J., Dubey, S., Salsburg, D.H. et al. (1978). Should there be statistical guidelines for medical research papers? *Biometrics* 34: 687–695.
51. Lo, B. (2015). Sharing clinical trial data: maximizing benefits, minimizing risk. *JAMA* 313: 793–794.
52. Taichman, D.B., Sahni, P., Pinborg, A. et al. (2017). Data sharing statements for clinical trials. *BMJ* https://doi.org/10.1136/bmj.c117.
53. Yancy, C.W., Harrington, R.A., and Bonow, R.O. (2018). Data sharing-the time has (not yet?) come. *JAMA Cardiol.* 3: 797–798.
54. Hamra, G.B., Goldstein, N.D., and Harper, S. (2019). Resource sharing to improve research quality. *J. Am. Heart Assoc.* https://doi.org/10.1161/JAHA.119.012292.
55. Longo, D.L. and Drazen, J.M. (2016). Data Sharing. *N. Engl. J. Med.* 374: 276–277.

56. Bauchner, H., Golub, R.M., and Fontanarosa, P.B. (2016). Data sharing: an ethical and scientific imperative. *JAMA* 315: 1237–1239.

57. Blomberg, N. and Lauer, K.B. (2020). Connecting data, tools and people across Europe: ELIXIR's response to the COVID-19 pandemic. *Eur. J. Hum. Genet.* 28: 719–723.

58. Rockhold, F., Nisen, P., and Freeman, A. (2016). Data sharing at a crossroads. *N. Engl. J. Med.* 375: 1115–1157.

59. Rockhold, F., Bromley, C., Wagner, E.K. et al. (2019). Open science: the open clinical trials data journey. *Clin. Trials* 16: 539–546.

60. Gibson, C.M. (2018). Moving from Hope to hard work in data sharing. *JAMA Cardiol.* 3: 795–796.

61. Boeckhout, M., Zielhuis, G.A., and Bredenoord, A.L. (2018). The FAIR guiding principles for data stewardship: fair enough? *Eur. J. Hum. Genet.* 26: 931–936.

62. Ohmann, C., Banzi, R., Canham, S. et al. (2107). Sharing and reuse of individual participant data from clinical trials: principles and recommendations. *BMJ Open* https://doi.org/10.1136/bmjopen-2017-018647.

63. Ross, J.S., Waldstreicher, J., Bamford, S. et al. (2018). Overview and experience of the YODA project with clinical trial data sharing after 5 years. *Sci. Data* https://doi.org/10.1038/sdata.2018.268.

64. Rowhani-Farid, A., Allen, M., and Barnett, A.G. (2017). What incentives increase data sharing in health and medical research? A systematic review. *Res. Integr. Peer Rev.* https://doi.org/10.1186/s41073-017-0028-9.

65. Nosek, B.A., Alter, G., Banks, G.C. et al. (2015). Promoting an open research culture. *Science* 348: 1422–1425.

66. Allen, C. and Mehler, D.M.A. (2019). Open science challenges, benefits and tips in early career and beyond. *PLoS Biol.* https://doi.org/10.1371/journal.pbio.3000587.

67. Mons, B. (2020). Invest 5% of research funds in ensuring data are reusable. *Nature* 578: 491.

68. Doshi, P., Dickersin, K., Healy, D. et al. (2013). Restoring invisible and abandoned trials: a call for people to publish the findings. *BMJ* https://doi.org/10.1136/bmj.f2865.

69. Doshi, P., Shamseer, L., Jones, M. et al. (2018). Restoring biomedical literature with RIAT. *BMJ* https://doi.org/10.1136/bmj.k1742.

70. Zhang, R. and Persaud, N. (2017). 8-way randomized controlled trial of Doxylamine, pyridoxine and Dicyclomine for nausea and vomiting during pregnancy: restoration of unpublished information. *PLoS One* https://doi.org/10.1371/journal.pone.0167609.

71. Persaud, N., Meaney, C., El-Emam, K. et al. (2018). Doxylamine-pyridoxine for nausea and vomiting of pregnancy randomized placebo controlled trial: Prespecified analyses and reanalysis. *PLoS One* https://doi.org/10.1371/journal.pone.0189978.

72. Le Noury, J., Nardo, J.M., Healy, D. et al. (2015). Restoring study 329: efficacy and harms of paroxetine and imipramine in treatment of major depression in adolescence. *BMJ* https://doi.org/10.1136/bmj.h4320.

73. Begg, C., Cho, M., Eastwood, S. et al. (1996). Improving the quality of reporting of randomized controlled trials. The CONSORT statement. *JAMA* 276: 637–639.

74. Schulz, K.F., Altman, D.G., and Moher, D. (2010). CONSORT 2010 statement: updated guidelines for reporting parallel group randomised trials. *BMJ* https://doi.org/10.1136/bmj.f4313.

75. Ghosn, L., Boutron, I., and Ravaud, P. (2019). Consolidated standards of reporting trials (CONSORT) extensions covered most types of randomized controlled trials, but the potential workload for authors was high. *J. Clin. Epidemiol.* 113: 168–175.

76. Wilson, B., Burnett, P., Moher, D. et al. (2018). Completeness of reporting of randomised controlled trials including people with transient ischaemic attack or stroke: a systematic review. *Eur. Stroke J.* 3: 337–346.

77. Yu, J., Li, X., Li, Y. et al. (2017). Quality of reporting in surgical randomized clinical trials. *Br. J. Surg.* 104: 296–303.

78. Dechartres, A., Trinquart, L., Atal, I. et al. (2017). Evolution of poor reporting and inadequate methods over time in 20 920 randomised controlled trials included in Cochrane reviews: research on research study. *BMJ* https://doi.org/10.1136/bmj.j2490.

79. Altman, D.G. (2005). Endorsement of the CONSORT statement by high impact medical journals: survey of instructions for authors. *BMJ* https://doi.org/10.1136/bmj.330.7499.1056.

80. Shamseer, L., Hopewell, S., Altman, D.G. et al. (2016). Update on the endorsement of CONSORT by high impact factor journals: a survey of journal "instructions to authors" in 2014. *Trials* https://doi.org/10.1186/s13063-016-1408-z.

81. Smith, T.A., Kulatilake, P., Brown, L.J. et al. (2015). Do surgery journals insist on reporting by CONSORT and PRISMA? A follow-up survey of 'instructions to authors'. *Ann. Med. Sur.* 4: 17–21.

82. Tetzlaff, J.M., Chan, A.W., Kitchen, J. et al. (2012). Guidelines for randomized clinical trial protocol content: a systematic review. *Syst. Rev.* https://doi.org/10.1186/2046-4053-1-43.

83. Chan, A.W., Tetzlaff, J.M., Altman, D.G. et al. (2013). SPIRIT 2013 statement: defining standard protocol items for clinical trials. *Ann. Intern. Med.* 158: 200–207.

84. Chan, A.W., Tetzlaff, J.M., Gotzsche, P.C. et al. (2013). SPIRIT 2013 explanation and elaboration: guidance for protocols of clinical trials. *BMJ* https://doi.org/10.1136/bmj.e7586.

85. Li, G., Abbade, L.P.F., Nwosu, I. et al. (2018). A systematic review of comparisons between protocols or registrations and full reports in primary biomedical research. *BMC Med. Res. Methodol.* https://doi.org/10.1186/s12874-017-0465-7.

86. Chan, A.-W. and Hrobjartsson, A. (2018). Promoting public access to clinical trial protocols: challenges and recommendations. *Trials* https://doi.org/10.1186/s13063-018-2510-1.

87. Lang, T. and Altman, D. (2016). Basic statistical reporting for articles published in clinical medical journals: the SAMPL guidelines. *Med. Writ.* 25: 31–36.

88. Ioannidis, J.P., Evans, S.J., Gotzsche, P.C. et al. (2004). Better reporting of harms in randomized trials: an extension of the CONSORT statement. *Ann. Intern. Med.* 141: 781–788.

89. Tang, E., Ravaud, P., Riveros, C. et al. (2015). Comparison of serious adverse events posted at http://ClinicalTrials.gov and published in corresponding journal articles. *BMC Med.* https://doi.org/10.1186/s12916-015-0430-4.

90. Favier, R. and Crepin, S. (2018). The reporting of harms in publications on randomized controlled trials funded by the "Programme

Hospitalier de Recherche Clinique," a French academic funding scheme. *Clin. Trials* 15: 257–267.

91. Hughes, S., Cohen, D., and Jaggi, R. (2014). Differences in reporting serious adverse events in industry sponsored clinical trial registries and journal articles on antidepressant and antipsychotic drugs: a cross-sectional study. *BMJ Open* https://doi.org/10.1136/bmjopen-2014-005535.

92. Golder, S., Loke, Y.K., Wright, K. et al. (2016). Reporting of adverse events in published and unpublished studies of health care interventions: a systematic review. *PLoS Med.* https://doi.org/10.1371/journal.pmed.1002127.

93. Hodkinson, A., Kirkham, J.J., Tudur-Smith, C. et al. (2013). Reporting of harms data in RCTs: a systematic review of empirical assessments against the CONSORT harms extension. *BMJ Open* https://doi.org/10.1136/bmjopen-2013-003436.

94. Goldacre, B., DeVito, N.J., Heneghan, C. et al. (2018). Compliance with requirement to report results on the EU clinical trials register: cohort study and web resource. *BMJ* https://doi.org/10.1136/bmj.k3218.

95. Moorthy, V.S., Karam, G., Vannice, K.S. et al. (2015). Rationale for WHO's new position calling for prompt reporting and public disclosure of interventional clinical trial results. *PLoS Med.* https://doi.org/10.1371/journal.pmed.1001819.

96. DeVito, N.J., Bacon, S., and Goldacre, B. (2020). Compliance with legal requirement to report clinical trial results on http://ClinicalTrials.gov: a cohort study. *Lancet* 395: 361–369.

97. Anderson, M.L., Chiswell, K., Peterson, E.D. et al. (2015). Compliance with results reporting at http://ClinicalTrials.gov. *N. Engl. J. Med.* 372: 1031–1039.

98. Weber, W.E., Merino, J.G., and Loder, E. (2015). Trial registration 10 years on. *BMJ* https://doi.org/10.1136/bmj.h3572.

99. Pansieri, C., Pandolfini, C., and Bonati, M. (2015). The evolution in registration of clinical trials: a chronicle of the historical calls and current initiatives promoting transparency. *Eur. J. Clin. Pharmacol.* 71: 1159–1164.

100. Zarin, D.A., Tse, T., Williams, R.J. et al. (2017). Update on trial registration 11 years after the ICMJE policy was established. *N. Engl. J. Med.* 376: 383–391.

101. Viergever, R.F. and Li, K. (2015). Trends in global clinical trial registration: an analysis of numbers of registered clinical trials in different parts of the world from 2004 to 2013. *BMJ Open* https://doi.org/10.1136/bmjopen-2015-008932.

102. Trinquart, L., Dunn, A.G., and Bourgeois, F.T. (2018). Registration of published randomized trials: a systematic review and meta-analysis. *BMC Med.* https://doi.org/10.1186/s12916-018-1168-6.

103. Dal-Re, R., Ross, J.S., and Marusic, A. (2016). Compliance with prospective trial registration guidance remained low in high-impact journals and has implications for primary end point reporting. *J. Clin. Epidemiol.* 75: 100–107.

104. Gopal, A.D., Wallach, J.D., Aminawung, J.A. et al. (2018). Adherence to the International Committee of Medical Journal Editors' (ICMJE) prospective registration policy and implications for outcome integrity: a cross-sectional analysis of trials published in high-impact specialty society journals. *Trials* https://doi.org/10.1186/s13063-018-2825-y.

105. Dechartres, A., Ravaud, P., Atal, I. et al. (2016). Association between trial registration and treatment effect estimates: a meta-epidemiological study. *BMC Med.* https://doi.org/10.1186/s12916-016-0639-x.

106. Papageorgiou, S.N., Xavier, G.M., Cobourne, M.T. et al. (2018). Registered trials report less beneficial treatment effects than unregistered ones: a meta-epidemiological study in orthodontics. *J. Clin. Epidemiol.* 100: 44–52.

107. Hunter, K.E., Seidler, A.L., and Askie, L.M. (2018). Prospective registration trends, reasons for retrospective registration and mechanisms to increase prospective registration compliance: descriptive analysis and survey. *BMJ Open* https://doi.org/10.1136/bmjopen-2017-019983.

108. Denneny, C., Bourne, S., and Kolstoe, S.E. (2019). Registration audit of clinical trials given a favourable opinion by UK

research ethics committees. *BMJ Open* https://doi.org/10.1136/bmjopen-2018-026840.

109. Liberati, A., Altman, D.G., Tetzlaff, J. et al. (2009). The PRISMA statement for reporting systematic reviews and meta-analyses of studies that evaluate healthcare interventions: explanation and elaboration. *J. Clin. Epidemiol.* https://doi.org/10.1016/j.jclinepi.2009.06.006.

110. Beller, E.M., Glasziou, P.P., Altman, D.G. et al. PRISMA for abstracts: reporting systematic reviews in journal and conference abstracts. *PLoS Med.* 2013 http://doi.org/10.1371/journal.pmed.1001419.

111. Zorzela, L., Loke, Y.K., Ioannidis, J.P. et al. (2016). PRISMA harms checklist: improving harms reporting in systematic reviews. *BMJ* https://doi.org/10.1136/bmj.i157.

112. Page, M.J. and Moher, D. (2017). Evaluations of the uptake and impact of the preferred reporting items for systematic reviews and meta-analyses (PRISMA) statement and extensions: a scoping review. *Syst. Rev.* https://doi.org/10.1186/s13643-017-0663-8.

113. Pussegoda, K., Turner, L., Garritty, C. et al. (2017). Systematic review adherence to methodological or reporting quality. *Syst. Rev.* https://doi.org/10.1186/s13643-017-0527-2.

114. Booth, A., Clarke, M., Dooley, G. et al. (2012). The nuts and bolts of PROSPERO: an international prospective register of systematic reviews. *Syst. Rev.* https://doi.org/10.1186/2046-4053-1-2.

115. Page, M.J., Shamseer, L., and Tricco, A.C. (2018). Registration of systematic reviews in PROSPERO: 30,000 records and counting. *Syst. Rev.* https://doi.org/10.1186/s13643-018-0699-4.

116. Moher, D., Shamseer, L., Clarke, M. et al. (2015). Preferred reporting items for systematic review and meta-analysis protocols (PRISMA-P) 2015 statement. *Syst. Rev.* https://doi.org/10.1186/2046-4053-4-1.

117. Shamseer, L., Moher, D., Clarke, M. et al. (2015). Preferred reporting items for systematic review and meta-analysis protocols (PRISMA-P) 2015: elaboration and explanation. *BMJ* https://doi.org/10.1136/bmj.g7647.

118. Niforatos, J.D., Weaver, M., and Johansen, M.E. (2019). Assessment of publication trends of systematic reviews and randomized clinical trials, 1995 to 2017. *JAMA Intern. Med.* 179: 1593–1594.

119. Sideri, S., Papageorgiou, S.N., and Eliades, T. (2018). Registration in the international prospective register of systematic reviews (PROSPERO) of systematic review protocols was associated with increased review quality. *J. Clin. Epidemiol.* 100: 103–110.

120. Ge, L., Tian, J.H., Li, Y.N. et al. (2018). Association between prospective registration and overall reporting and methodological quality of systematic reviews: a meta-epidemiological study. *J. Clin. Epidemiol.* 93: 45–55.

121. Allers, K., Hoffmann, F., Mathes, T. et al. (2018). Systematic reviews with published protocols compared to those without: more effort, older search. *J. Clin. Epidemiol.* 95: 102–110.

122. Tricco, A.C., Cogo, E., Page, M.J. et al. (2016). A third of systematic reviews changed or did not specify the primary outcome: a PROSPERO register study. *J. Clin. Epidemiol.* 79: 46–54.

123. Delgado, A.F. and Delgado, A.F. (2017). Inconsistent reporting between meta-analysis protocol and publication – a cross-sectional study. *Anticancer Res.* 37: 5101–5107.

124. Koensgen, N., Rombey, T., Allers, K. et al. (2019). Comparison of non-Cochrane systematic reviews and their published protocols: differences occurred frequently but were seldom explained. *J. Clin. Epidemiol.* 110: 34–41.

125. Altman, D.G. and Simera, I. (2016). A history of the evolution of guidelines for reporting medical research: the long road to the EQUATOR network. *J. R. Soc. Med.* 109: 67–77.

126. Samaan, Z., Mhuagbaw, L., Kosa, D. et al. (2013). A systematic scoping review of adherence to reporting guidelines in health care literature. *J. Multidiscip. Healthc.* 6: 169–188.

127. Blanco, D., Altman, D., Moher, D. et al. (2019). Scoping review on interventions to improve adherence to reporting guidelines in health research. *BMJ Open* https://doi.org/10.1136/bmjopen-2018-026589.

128. Hopewell, S., Boutron, I., Altman, D. et al. (2016). Impact of a web-based tool (WebCONSORT) to improve the reporting of randomised trials: results of a randomised controlled trial. *BMC Med.* https://doi.org/10.1186/s12916-016-0736-x.

129. Blanco, D., Schroter, S., Aldcroft, A. et al. (2020). Effect of an editorial intervention to improve the completeness of reporting of randomised trials: a randomised controlled trial. *BMJ Open* https://doi.org/10.1136/bmjopen-2020-036799.

130. Moher, D. and Altman, D.G. (2015). Four proposals to help improve the medical research literature. *PLoS Med.* https://doi.org/10.1371/journal.pmed.1001864.

131. Krummel, M., Blish, C., Kuhns, M. et al. (2019). Universal principled review: a community-driven method to improve peer review. *Cell* 179: 1441–1445.

132. Hames, I. (2014). Peer review at the beginning of the 21st century. *Sci. Ed.* 1: 4–8.

133. Heneghan, C. and McCartney, M. (2019). Declaring interests and restoring trust in medicine. *BMJ* https://doi.org/10.1136/bmj.d7202.

134. Kaelin, W.G. Jr. (2017). Publish houses of brick, not mansions of straw. *Nature* 545: 387.

135. Weston, J., Dwan, K., Altman, D. et al. (2016). Feasibility study to examine discrepancy rates in prespecified and reported outcomes in articles submitted to the BMJ. *BMJ Open* https://doi.org/10.1136/bmjopen-2015-010075.

136. Wicherts, J.M. (2017). The weak spots in contemporary science (and how to fix them). *Animals* https://doi.org/10.3390/ani7120090.

137. Clark, L., Fairhurst, C., and Torgerson, D.J. (2016). Allocation concealment in randomised controlled trials: are we getting better? *BMJ* https://doi.org/10.1136/bmj.i5663.

138. Simmons, J.P., Nelson, L.D., and Simonsohn, U. (2011). False-positive psychology: undisclosed flexibility in data collection and analysis allows presenting anything as significant. *Psychol. Sci.* 22: 1359–1366.

139. Cobo, E., Selva-O'Callagham, A., Ribera, J.M. et al. (2007). Statistical reviewers improve reporting in biomedical articles: a randomized trial. *PLoS One* https://doi.org/10.1371/journal.pone.0000332.

140. Dexter, F. and Shafer, S.L. (2017). Narrative review of statistical reporting checklists, mandatory statistical editing, and rectifying common problems in the reporting of scientific articles. *Anesth. Analg.* 124: 943–947.

141. Woznyj, H.M., Grenier, K., Ross, R. et al. (2018). Results-blind review: a masked crusader for science. *Eur. J. Work Organ. Psychol.* 27: 561–576.

142. Editorial (2019). In praise of process. *Nature* 571: 447.

143. Wilkinson, J., Pellicer, A., and Niederberger, C. (2019). Registered reports: prospective peer review emphasizes science over spin. *Fertil. Steril.* 111: 831–832.

144. Adam, D. (2019). Reproducibility trial publishes two conclusions for one paper. *Nature* 570: 16.

145. Avidan, M.S., Ioannidis, J.P.A., and Mashour, G.A. (2019). Independent discussion sections for improving inferential reproducibility in published research. *Br. J. Anaesth.* 122: 413–420.

146. Sneyd, J.R. (2019). Who watches the watchmen and the problem of recursive flea bites. *Br. J. Anaesth.* 122: 407–408.

147. Malcom, D. (2018). It's time we fix the peer review system. *Am. J. Pharm. Educ.* 82: 385–387.

148. Zietman, A.L. (2017). The ethics of scientific publishing: black, White, and "fifty shades of gray". *Int. J. Radiat. Oncol. Biol. Phys.* 99: 275–279.

149. Rajpert-De Meyts, E., Losito, S., and Carrell, D.T. (2016). Rewarding peer-review work: the Publons initiative. *Andrology* 4: 985–986.

150. Smith, D.R. (2016). Will Publons popularize the scientific peer-review process? *Bioscience* 66: 265–266.

151. da Silva, J.A.T., Al-Khatib, A., and Dobranszki, J. (2017). Fortifying the corrective nature of post-publication peer review: identifying weaknesses, use of journal clubs, and rewarding conscientious behavior. *Sci. Eng. Ethics* 23: 1213–1226.

152. Goldacre, B. (2015). How to get all trials reported: audit, better data, and individual accountability. *PLoS Med.* https://doi.org/10.1371/journal.pmed.1001821.

153. DeVito, N.J., Bacon, S., and Goldacre, B. (2019). FDAAA TrialsTracker: a live informatics tool to monitor compliance with

FDA requirements to report clinical trial results. *bioRxiv* https://doi.org/10.1101/266452.

154. Kolstoe, S.E., Shanahan, D.R., and Wisely, J. (2017). Should research ethics committees police reporting bias? *BMJ* https://doi.org/10.1136/bmj.j1501.

155. Dal-Re, R. and Marusic, A. (2016). Prevention of selective outcome reporting: let us start from the beginning. *Eur. J. Clin. Pharmacol.* 72: 1283–1288.

156. Kahan, B.C. and Jairath, V. (2018). Outcome pre-specification requires sufficient detail to guard against outcome switching in clinical trials: a case study. *Trials* https://doi.org/10.1186/s13063-018-2654-z.

157. Ioannidis, J.P., Caplan, A.L., and Dal-Re, R. (2017). Outcome reporting bias in clinical trials: why monitoring matters. *BMJ* https://doi.org/10.1136/bmj.j408.

158. Dal-Re, R. and Caplan, A.L. (2015). Journal editors impasse with outcome reporting bias. *Eur. J. Clin. Investig.* 45: 895–898.

159. van der Steen, J.T., Ter Riet, G., van den Bogert, C.A. et al. (2019). Causes of reporting bias: a theoretical framework. *F1000Res.* https://doi.org/10.12688/f1000research.18310.2.

160. Greenberg, L., Jairath, V., Pearse, R. et al. (2018). Pre-specification of statistical analysis approaches in published clinical trial protocols was inadequate. *J. Clin. Epidemiol.* 101: 53–60.

161. Rawlinson, C. and Bloom, T. (2019). New preprint server for medical research. *BMJ* https://doi.org/10.1136/bmj.l2301.

162. Oakden-Rayner, L., Beam, A.L., and Palmer, L.J. (2018). Medical journals should embrace preprints to address the reproducibility crisis. *Int. J. Epidemiol.* 47: 1363–1365.

163. Johansson, M.A., Reich, N.G., Meyers, L.A. et al. (2018). Preprints: an underutilized mechanism to accelerate outbreak science. *PLoS Med.* https://doi.org/10.1371/journal.pmed.1002549.

164. Majumder, M.S. and Mandl, K.D. (2020). Early in the epidemic: impact of preprints on global discourse about COVID-19 transmissibility. *Lancet* 8: e627–e630.

165. Bauchner, H. (2017). The rush to publication: an editorial and scientific mistake. *JAMA* 318: 1109–1110.

166. Tabor, E. (2016). Prepublication culture in clinical research. *Lancet* 387: 750.

167. Mercier, M., Magloire, V., and Karnani, M. (2020). Enhancing scientific dissemination in neuroscience via preprint peer-review: "peer community in circuit neuroscience". *Neuroanat. Behav.* 2: 1–5.

168. Skoric, L., Glasnovic, A., and Petrak, J. (2020). A publishing pandemic during the COVID-19 pandemic: how challenging can it become? *Croat. Med. J.* 61: 79–81.

169. Horton, R. (2002). Postpublication criticism and the shaping of clinical knowledge. *JAMA* 287: 2843–2847.

170. Goldacre, B., Drysdale, H., Dale, A. et al. (2019). COMPare: a prospective cohort study correcting and monitoring 58 misreported trials in real time. *Trials* https://doi.org/10.1186/s13063-019-3173-2.

171. Gotzsche, P.C., Delamothe, T., Godlee, F. et al. (2010). Adequacy of authors' replies to criticism raised in electronic letters to the editor: cohort study. *BMJ* https://doi.org/10.1136/bmj.i5239.

172. Rogers, J.R., Mills, H., Grossman, L.V. et al. (2019). Understanding the nature and scope of clinical research commentaries in PubMed. *J. Am. Med. Inform. Assoc.* 27: 449–456.

173. Knoepfler, P. (2015). Reviewing post-publication peer review. *Trends Genet.* 31: 221–223.

174. Horbach, S. and Halffman, W.W. (2018). The changing forms and expectations of peer review. *Res. Integr. Peer Rev.* https://doi.org/10.1186/s41073-018-0051-5.

175. Peterson, G.I. (2018). Postpublication peer review: a crucial tool. *Science* 359: 1225–1226.

176. Jefferson, T. (2018), P D: RIP PubMed commons. https://blogs.bmj.com/bmj/2018/02/21/tom-jefferson-and-peter-doshi-rip-pubmed-commons. Accessed 6 February 2020.

177. Price, A.R. (2013). Research misconduct and its federal regulation: the origin and history of the Office of Research Integrity – with personal views by ORI's former associate director for investigative oversight. *Account Res.* 20: 291–319.

178. Anderson, M.S. (2014). Global research integrity in relation to the United States' research-integrity infrastructure. *Account Res.* 21: 1–8.

179. Resnik, D.B. and Shamoo, A.E. (2011). The Singapore statement on research integrity. *Account Res.* 18: 71–75.

180. Bouter, L.M. (2018). Fostering responsible research practices is a shared responsibility of multiple stakeholders. *J. Clin. Epidemiol.* 96: 143–146.

181. Resnik, D.B. and Dinse, G.E. (2012). Do U.S. research institutions meet or exceed federal mandates for instruction in responsible conduct of research? A national survey. *Acad. Med.* 87: 1237–1242.

182. Schoenherr, J. and Williams-Jones, B. (2011). Research integrity/misconduct policies of Canadian universities. *Can. J. High. Educ.* 41: 1–17.

183. Khajuria, A. and Agha, R. (2014). Fraud in scientific research – birth of the concordat to uphold research integrity in the United Kingdom. *J. R. Soc. Med.* 107: 61–65.

184. Tavare, A. (2011). Managing research misconduct: is anyone getting it right? *BMJ* https://doi.org/10.1136/bmj.d8212.

185. Godecharle, S., Nemery, B., and Dierickx, K. (2013). Guidance on research integrity: no union in Europe. *Lancet* 381: 1097–1098.

186. Torjesen, I. (2012). Strategy for boosting integrity of research is launched in UK. *BMJ* https://doi.org/10.1136/bmj.e4747.

187. Bonn, N.A., Godecharle, S., and Dierickx, K. (2017). European Universities' guidance on research integrity and misconduct: accessibility, approaches, and content. *J. Empir. Res. Hum. Res. Ethics* 12: 33–44.

188. Steneck, N.H. (2013). Research ethics. Global research integrity training. *Science* 340: 552–553.

189. Godecharle, S., Nemery, B., and Dierickx, K. (2014). Heterogeneity in European research integrity guidance: relying on values or norms? *J. Empir. Res. Hum. Res. Ethics* 9: 79–90.

190. Forsberg, E.M., Anthun, F.O., Bailey, S. et al. (2018). Working with research integrity-guidance for research performing organisations: the Bonn PRINTEGER statement. *Sci. Eng. Ethics* 24: 1023–1034.

191. Zwart, H. and Ter Meulen, R. (2019). Addressing research integrity challenges: from penalising individual perpetrators to fostering research ecosystem quality care. *Life Sci. Soc. Policy* 15: 5.

192. Editorial (2009). Teaching responsible conduct of research. *Lancet* 374: 1568.

193. Titus, S. and Bosch, X. (2010). Tie funding to research integrity. *Nature* 466: 436–437.

194. Shaw, D.M. and Erren, T.C. (2015). Ten simple rules for protecting research integrity. *PLoS Comput. Biol.* https://doi.org/10.1371/journal.pcbi.1004388.

195. Kalichman, M. (2014). Rescuing responsible conduct of research (RCR) education. *Account Res.* 21: 68–83.

196. Gunsalus, C.K. and Robinson, A.D. (2018). Nine pitfalls of research misconduct. *Nature* 557: 297–299.

197. Plemmons, D.K. and Kalichman, M.W. (2018). Mentoring for responsible research: the creation of a curriculum for faculty to teach RCR in the research environment. *Sci. Eng. Ethics* 24: 207–226.

198. Marusic, A., Wager, E., Utrobicic, A. et al. (2016). Interventions to prevent misconduct and promote integrity in research and publication. *Cochrane Database Syst. Rev.* http://doi.org/10.1002/14651858.MR000038.pub2.

199. Kalichman, M. (2013). A brief history of RCR education. *Account Res.* 20: 380–394.

200. Bruton, S.V., Medlin, M., Brown, M. et al. (2020). Personal motivations and systemic incentives: scientists on questionable research practices. *Sci. Eng. Ethics* 26: 1531–1547.

201. Bruton, S.V., Brown, M., Sacco, D.F. et al. (2019). Testing an active intervention to deter researchers' use of questionable research practices. *Res. Integr. Peer Rev.* https://doi.org/10.1186/s41073-019-0085-3.

202. Satalkar, P. and Shaw, D. (2018). Is failure to raise concerns about misconduct a breach of integrity? Researchers' reflections on reporting misconduct. *Account. Res.* 25: 311–339.

203. Andersen, J.R., Byrjalsen, I., Bihlet, A. et al. (2015). Impact of source data verification on data quality in clinical trials: an empirical post

hoc analysis of three phase 3 randomized clinical trials. *Br. J. Clin. Pharmacol.* 79: 660–668.

204. Morrison, B.W., Cochran, C.J., White, J.G. et al. (2011). Monitoring the quality of conduct of clinical trials: a survey of current practices. *Clin. Trials* 8: 342–349.

205. Olsen, R., Bihlet, A.R., Kalakou, F. et al. (2016). The impact of clinical trial monitoring approaches on data integrity and cost – a review of current literature. *Eur. J. Clin. Pharmacol.* 72: 399–412.

206. Buyse, M., George, S.L., Evans, S. et al. (1999). The role of biostatistics in the prevention, detection and treatment of fraud in clinical trials. *Stat. Med.* 18: 3435–3451.

207. Trotta, L., Kabeya, Y., Buyse, M. et al. (2019). Detection of atypical data in multicenter clinical trials using unsupervised statistical monitoring. *Clin. Trials* 16: 512–522.

208. Knepper, D., Lindblad, A.S., Sharma, G. et al. (2016). Statistical monitoring in clinical trials: best practices for detecting data anomalies suggestive of fabrication or misconduct. *Ther. Innov. Regul. Sci.* 50: 144–154.

209. Tijdink, J.K., Bouter, L.M., Veldkamp, C.L. et al. (2016). Personality traits are associated with research misbehavior in Dutch scientists: a cross-sectional study. *PLoS One* https://doi.org/10.1371/journal.pone.0163251.

210. Pryor, E.R., Habermann, B., and Broome, M.E. (2007). Scientific misconduct from the perspective of research coordinators: a national survey. *J. Med. Ethics* 33: 365–369.

211. Bouter, L.M. and Hendrix, S. (2017). Both whistleblowers and the scientists they accuse are vulnerable and deserve protection. *Account Res.* 24: 359–366.

212. Resnik, D.B. and Shamoo, A.E. (2017). Fostering research integrity. *Account Res.* 24: 367–372.

213. Chordiya, R., Sabharwal, M., Relly, J.E. et al. (2020). Organizational protection for whistleblowers: a cross-national study. *Public Manag. Rev.* 22: 527–552.

214. Millar, N., Salager-Meyer, F., and Budgell, B. (2019). "It is important to reinforce the importance of . . .": 'hype' in reports of randomized controlled trials. *Engl. Specif. Purp.* 54: 139–151.

215. Caulfield, T. (2018). Spinning the genome: why science hype matters. *Perspect. Biol. Med.* 61: 560–571.

216. Boutron, I. and Ravaud, P. (2018). Misrepresentation and distortion of research in biomedical literature. *Proc. Natl. Acad. Sci. U. S. A.* 115: 2613–2619.

217. Chiu, K., Grundy, Q., and Bero, L. (2017). 'Spin' in published biomedical literature: a methodological systematic review. *PLoS Biol.* https://doi.org/10.1371/journal.pbio.2002173.

218. Hopf, H., Matlin, S.A., Mehta, G. et al. (2020). Blocking the hype-hypocrisy-falsification-fakery pathway is needed to safeguard science. *Angew. Chem. Int. Ed.* 59: 2150–2154.

219. Shawwa, K., Kallas, R., Koujanian, S. et al. (2016). Requirements of clinical journals for Authors' disclosure of financial and non-financial conflicts of interest: a cross sectional study. *PLoS One* https://doi.org/10.1371/journal.pone.0152301.

220. Khamis, A.M., Hakoum, M.B., Bou-Karroum, L. et al. (2017). Requirements of health policy and services journals for authors to disclose financial and non-financial conflicts of interest: a cross-sectional study. *Health Res. Policy Syst.* https://doi.org/10.1186/s12961-017-0244-2.

221. Bauchner, H., Fontanarosa, P.B., and Flanagin, A. (2018). Conflicts of interests, authors, and journals new challenges for a persistent problem. *JAMA* 320: 2315–2318.

222. Cherla, D.V., Olavarria, O.A., Holihan, J.L. et al. (2017). Discordance of conflict of interest self-disclosure and the centers of Medicare and Medicaid services. *J. Surg. Res.* 218: 18–22.

223. Menkes, D.B., Masters, J.D., Broring, A. et al. (2018). What does 'Unpaid Consultant' signify? A survey of euphemistic language in conflict of interest declarations. *J. Gen. Intern. Med.* 33: 139–141.

224. Lichter, A.S. and McKinney, R. (2012). Toward a harmonized and centralized conflict of interest disclosure: progress from an IOM initiative. *JAMA* 308: 2093–2094.

225. Dunn, A.G., Coiera, E., Mandl, K.D. et al. (2016). Conflict of interest disclosure in biomedical research: a review of current practices, biases, and the role of public registries in improving transparency. *Res. Integr. Peer Rev.* https://doi.org/10.1186/s41073-016-0006-7.

226. Tereskerz, P. and Mills, A. (2012). COI policies: tax dollars should not be used to fund U.S. institutions not making the grade. *Account Res.* 19: 243–246.

227. Richman, V. and Richman, A. (2012). A tale of two perspectives: regulation versus self-regulation. A financial reporting approach (from Sarbanes-Oxley) for research ethics. *Sci. Eng. Ethics* 18: 241–246.

228. Abbott, A. (2019). The integrity inspectors. *Nature* 575: 430–433.

229. Dyer, C. (2013). Bioanalyst gets jail sentence for falsifying preclinical trial data. *BMJ* https://doi.org/10.1136/bmj.f2514.

230. Tilden, S.J. (2010). Incarceration, restitution, and lifetime debarment: legal consequences of scientific misconduct in the Eric Poehlman case: commentary on: "scientific forensics: how the office of research integrity can assist institutional investigations of research misconduct during oversight review". *Sci. Eng. Ethics* 16: 737–741.

231. Dyer, O. (2016). Australian neuroscientist given two year suspended sentence for falsifying Parkinson's research. *BMJ* https://doi.org/10.1136/bmj.i2013.

232. Sovacool, B.K. (2005). Using criminalization and due process to reduce scientific misconduct. *Am. J. Bioeth.* 5: W1–W7.

233. Collier, R. (2015). Scientific misconduct or criminal offence? *CMAJ* 187: 1273–1274.

234. Adams, D. and Pimple, K.D. (2005). Research misconduct and crime lessons from criminal science on preventing misconduct and promoting integrity. *Account Res.* 12: 225–240.

235. AllTrials Campaign (2019). http://www.alltrials.net Accessed 20 November 2019.

236. Strech, D., Weissgerber, T., and Dirnagl, U. (2020). Improving the trustworthiness, usefulness, and ethics of biomedical research through an innovative and comprehensive institutional initiative. *PLoS Biol.* https://doi.org/10.1371/journal.pbio.3000576.

237. Anonymous: The REWARD Campaign. *The Lancet.* https://www.thelancet.com/campaigns/efficiency (accessed 7 May 2020).

Index

A

abandoned trials 43, 44–45, 129, 171, 197
abstracts, misleading 116
acne and jelly baby consumption 69
adequacy of sources 84–85
adverse events
  meta-analysis 89
  reporting 24, 199
allocation
  methodology development 8–12
  randomisation 8–10, 19–21
  subversion 20–21
AllTrials campaign 215–216
alternate allocation 9
alternate forms of peer review 205–206
alternate selection 8
analytical bias 64–80
  covariate selection 70–71
  data exclusions 68
  hypothesising after the results are known 68
  multiple comparisons 68–69
  p-values 65–67, 113, 183–184
  research practices 67–71
  statistical analysis plans 71–72
  subgroup analyses 69–70
angina 11
animal magnetism 11
aspirin 4

assessment of outcomes 22–28
  analytical bias 64–80, 183–184
  averages vs. individuals 51
  COMET Initiative 49
  composite outcomes 47–49
  covariate selection 70–71
  data exclusions 68
  data quality monitoring 212–213
  hypothesising after the results are known 68
  low power 29–30
  misleading/weak evidence 51–53
  missing data 26–28, 49–51, 92–93
  monitoring selective reporting 164
  multiple comparisons 68–69
  patient characteristics 50
  primary outcome switching 22–23
  p-values 65–67, 113, 183–184
  SAMPL Guidelines 199
  selective reporting 164, 207–208
  small samples 28–30
  spin 115–117, 165
  statistical analysis plans 71–72
  subgroup analyses 69–70
  surrogate outcomes 31, 46–47
assessment of research *see* auditing; peer review; research assessment
astrological signs 69
auditing 207, 214–215
availability of expertise 169

Evidence in Medicine: The Common Flaws, Why They Occur and How to Prevent Them, First Edition. Iain K Crombie.
© 2021 John Wiley & Sons Ltd. Published 2021 by John Wiley & Sons Ltd.